Wellbeing for Veterinarians and the Veterinary Team

Wellbeing for Veterinarians and the Veterinary Team

Edited by

Carrie Jurney, DVM, DACVIM (Neurology)
Not One More Vet, Inc
San Francisco, CA
USA

Tracy Witte, PhD
Department of Psychological Sciences
Auburn University
Auburn, Al
USA

WILEY

Published by John Wiley & Sons, Inc., Hoboken, New Jersey.

Library of Congress Cataloging-in-Publication Data applied for:

Paperback ISBN: 9781394220717

Cover Design: Wiley
Cover Images: Inset photo: Courtney Phillips, RVT and Carrie Jurney; Background Image: Bruce Francke, DVM

Set in 9.5/12pt STIXTwoText by Straive, Pondicherry, India

Printed and bound by CPI Group (UK) Ltd, Croydon, CR0 4YY

C9781394220717_230726

In dedication to Dr. David Bartram, who showed me that science could be a path to happiness, and to Dr. Nicole McArthur, founder of Not One More Vet, who, in her desire for connection, sparked a global movement for the wellbeing of her community.

Contents

List of Contributors

Elisabeth Cavallaro, MPH, MCHES
American Association of Veterinary Medical Colleges
Washington, DC
USA

Malissa Clark, PhD
Department of Pyschology
University of Georgia
Athens, GA
USA

Lisa M. Greenhill, MPA, EdD
American Association of Veterinary Medical Colleges
Washington, DC
USA

Meredith Jones, DVM, CSLP®, AFC®
Allvet Financial
Richmond, VA
USA

Carrie Jurney, DVM, DACVIM (Neurology)
Not One More Vet, Inc
San Francisco, CA
USA

Olivia Knizek, PhD, CMPC
Student Health & Counseling Services
University of California Davis
Davis, CA
USA

Lori Kogan, PhD
Colorado State University
College of Veterinary Medicine and Biomedical Sciences
Fort Collins, CO
USA

Sharon Kramper, PhD
Northwestern University Feinberg School of Medicine
Chicago, IL
USA

Katie Lawlor, Psy.D
Not One More Vet, Inc
San Francisco, CA
USA

Jesse S. Michel, PhD
Department of Psychological Sciences
Auburn University
Auburn, AL
USA

Sraavya Polisetti
American Association of Veterinary Medical Colleges
Washington, DC
USA

Skylar Oney, MS
Department of Pyschology
University of Georgia
Athens, GA
USA

Zachary Ward, PhD
School of Veterinary Medicine
University of California Davis
Davis, CA
USA

Tracy Witte, PhD
Department of Psychological Sciences
Auburn University
Auburn, AL
USA

Foreword

If you work in veterinary medicine, you know that there are few professions where love and loss sit so closely together, so often, in a single day. In a single shift you might celebrate a new puppy, stabilize a crashing patient, translate complicated diagnostics into human language, and then guide someone through the final moments with the animal who has been their best friend for 15 years. You move between joy and grief with breathtaking speed, all while the phone keeps ringing and the next case is already waiting. You hold science in one hand and heartbreak in the other, and you keep showing up.

I have had the privilege of working in veterinary medicine for more than 20 years as a social worker, and I helped build veterinary social work as a practice space within the profession. Very quickly after my feet hit the clinical floor, I realized that veterinary hospitals function much like human hospitals: high stakes, rapid decisions, tight teams, and ethical complexity. What surprised me most, though, was not the similarity – it was the compassion. I was struck by how hardworking veterinarians are, how self-sacrificing they can be, and how deeply they love the animals in their care. I often say I learned more about compassion from veterinary medicine than my own profession, social work.

This new volume on veterinary well-being is edited by two women I trust deeply: Dr. Carrie Jurney, DVM, and Dr. Tracy Witte, PhD. I met them both at AVMA Wellbeing Roundtables and had the immediate, unmistakable sense that we would have long-standing and meaningful professional relationships. It's rare to meet leaders who can sit with the raw truth of this work – and then organize, research, advocate, and build to support it.

Carrie is a stalwart and wonderful leader for veterinary medicine. Through her leadership with Not One More Vet (NOMV), she has helped create pathways for connection, education, and support in a profession where too many have felt alone. Tracy is a grounded and trustworthy scholar who brings essential science to the often emotional question of suicidality in veterinary medicine. She has helped our community move beyond rumor, shame, and "we don't talk about that," toward clearer understanding and more actionable prevention.

For nearly a decade, it has been an honor to work alongside both of them, including in the development of Lifeboat by NOMV. I think of Lifeboat as a compassionate response to a simple truth: isolation makes suffering louder. Peer support does not replace therapy or clinical care, and it does not pretend to. But it can be the difference between "I'm alone with this" and "someone understands," and that difference can keep a person tethered to life and to community. That spirit – honest, practical, and deeply human – runs through this book.

This book arrives in a moment when veterinary medicine is telling the truth about the costs and benefits of being in the profession "out loud." The work veterinary professionals love can also come at a cost. Research continues to document stress, burnout, and psychological distress across veterinary team, and multiple studies have shown elevated suicide risk among veterinarians (and, in some studies, veterinary technicians) compared with the general population. The unique realities of veterinary workplaces – including access to lethal means – make prevention both urgent and nuanced.

Happily, the story of veterinary well-being is not only a story of risk. It is also a story of meaning – of moral courage, deep connection, and everyday acts of care that make veterinary medicine a very "tight knit community." Many veterinary professionals have had a call to profession for as long as they can remember! That sense of purpose can be a powerful protective factor, but only when it is supported by environments that make sustainable caring possible.

One of the strengths of this volume is its breadth and realism. The chapters move from the foundations of well-being to the forces that shape it: the individual, diversity and belonging, mental health, suicidality in veterinary medicine, professional stressors, workplace culture, finances, burnout, and the science of positive psychology. The table of contents reads like a map of the terrain veterinary professionals actually walk – inner experience and external systems, personal practices and organizational responsibility. Just as importantly, the author team is interdisciplinary, bringing veterinary expertise into conversation with psychology, research, coaching, and applied well-being science.

I am especially grateful that this book refuses to turn resilience into a moral test. Resilience is not rugged individualism. Well-being is not a reward you earn after you prove you can survive. Yes, individual skills matter: recovery practices, emotional regulation, self-awareness, connection, counseling, and medical care when needed, and the ability to ask for help early rather than late. But individual skills cannot compensate for chronic overload, economic pressure, or cultures that normalize the impossible. We need personal tools and system change – together.

That brings me to a small confession. Every time a veterinarian sets a boundary – says no, protects a day off, asks for coverage, takes a mental health appointment, joins a peer-support space, or stops normalizing the unsustainable – I have a little cheerleader inside of me who is happily bubbling over. Not because boundaries are easy, and not because they fix everything, but because they are acts of self care and integrity. In a caregiving profession, boundaries are not selfish, they are an ethical responsibility.

So as you read, approach these pages the way you approach a complex case: with curiosity, compassion, and a willingness to try what it takes to heal. If you are a student or new graduate, let this book shape your habits and language before burnout becomes your teacher. If you are a technician, assistant, client service representative, practice manager, or support staff member, I hope you feel seen here – well-being is a team reality, not a "doctor issue." If you lead, use this book as a blueprint for building conditions where people can do excellent work without sacrificing themselves.

I believe this volume will provide valuable information to help you stay connected to what called you to veterinary medicine. May it strengthen your capacity to care for others without abandoning yourself.

Elizabeth B. Strand, PhD, LCSW
Founding Director, Veterinary Social Work
University of Tennessee College of Veterinary Medicine

Acknowledgments

To my co-author, Dr. Tracy Witte. Thank you for being the balance to my chaos. I appreciate your dedication, your organization, and your patience more than you know. Truly, this book would not exist without you.

To Maya Ruffino, LCSW and Dr. Michelle Guchereau, for their enduring support of my personal wellbeing.

To my dear friend Michael, who, when I asked if I should really take on a textbook while I was starting a practice, sagely answered: "We both know you are going to do it, so let's skip to the part where you are complaining about how busy you are." How dare you know me so well, sir.

To the volunteers, staff, and community members of Not One More Vet, especially the founding board members: Nicole, David, Jason and Melanie. As hard as those early days were, I hope we can all look back at what we accomplished with pride.

To Dr. Elizabeth Strand, I will be eternally grateful to the universe for bringing us together at that committee meeting. I would sit through a thousand more boring, bureaucratic meetings if I knew our friendship was at the end. Thank you so much for your curiosity, intelligence, your kindness, your passion, and most of all, your friendship. To my husband, Chris, for his endless patience with my never-ending projects and for being my living proof of what this book keeps coming back to: that family and strong relationships are a cornerstone of wellbeing. You are the foundation that makes all of this possible.

CARRIE JURNEY

I first want to acknowledge Carrie for inviting me to join her on this book-writing adventure. We may have each lost part of a finger along the way (true story), but look at what we've managed to accomplish! Thank you also to Elizabeth Strand for introducing me to Carrie and for being such a wonderful collaborator and "yin" to my "yang."

Second, I want to acknowledge the thousands of veterinarians, veterinary technicians, and veterinary students who have contributed to my research studies over the years. I never anticipated that veterinary well-being would become a major focus of my career, but your enthusiasm and passion for improving mental health and preventing suicide have been supremely motivating.

Third, I want to acknowledge each and every one of my PhD students, past and present, for inspiring me to look at things in new ways and keeping me young (while occasionally causing me to sprout new gray hairs). Thank you, Maggie Davis, Kelly Zuromski, Jami Gauthier, Ian

Cero, Caitlin Williams, Liz Spitzer, Eric Crosby, Sharon Kramper, Sydney Waitz-Kudla, Cassidy Brydon Chesnutt, Hailey Fox Mumma, Hannah Sawyer, Marielle Gomez, and Aishwarya Chowdhary. Thank you also to my incredible colleagues, especially Nadia Bhuiyan, Tiffany Brown, Chris Correia, and Jonathan Kunstman, who have made the Auburn University Department of Psychological Sciences an ideal academic home for me.

Fourth, I want to acknowledge my academic siblings who have served as an irreplaceable circle of trust over the past two decades. Thank you, April Smith, Kim Van Orden, Katie Gordon, and Jill Holm-Denoma; I truly could not be doing this job without you.

Fifth, I want to acknowledge my mentors, who have shaped my professional development in innumerable ways. Thank you, Thomas Joiner and Frank Weathers. Everything I write today has been shaped by your feedback.

Sixth, I want to acknowledge my family. Mom, Dad, Jamie, and Annie, thank you for your unending support and cheerleading over the years. Seth and Sidney Rose, thank you for giving me the best reasons to leave my work behind at the end of the day and run home to you.

Finally, I want to extend my deepest gratitude to Dr. Pete Marine and his team at East University Veterinary Hospital in Auburn, Alabama. Y'all are the medical providers I've had the longest relationship with in my life, and you've seen me at my highest when welcoming new dogs and cats into the family and at my lowest when we have to inevitably say goodbye. You are constantly on my mind when engaging in this work.

TRACY WITTE

Introduction

CHAPTER 1

Carrie Jurney, DVM, DACVIM (Neurology)

Not One More Vet, Inc, San Francisco, CA, USA

In veterinary medicine, we discuss "quality of life" a great deal. Improving and protecting the quality of life for our patients is a primary driver of our work lives. At the most basic level, adequate quality of life entails the ability to perform basic bodily functions (breathing, eating, drinking, etc.) without distress or physical pain. However, life, and all that it entails, has a much broader experience than those checkboxes. A life, be it of an animal or a person, contains a multitude of experiences, both positive and negative. The goal of a helping profession like ours is to help minimize the negative and maximize the positive. The particulars of what that entails will vary deeply from animal to animal and from person to person.

A single negative does not necessarily override the positives. Clients will often fixate on physical pain in quality-of-life discussions, even if it's relatively minor. Perhaps a completely pain-free life is not a possibility for that patient. However, depending on the severity, it may not be enough to override positive aspects of the patient's life. I often tell these clients, "Look, I have a bad ankle. It hurts from time to time, and I can't be a distance runner anymore, but I hardly think it's a reason to put me down." Similarly, a single positive does not override other negatives. For instance, clients will also focus on the fact that a pet is still eating, even though objectively, the rest of their life has little positive. A surgeon colleague, Dr. Sharon Gottfried, has told many a Labrador owner that those dogs will "continue to eat two weeks after they have died," and therefore, by itself, appetite is not an appropriate measure of quality of life for these patients. Even within the basic quality-of-life checkboxes, there is a great deal of gray area in discussions of what a happy life entails.

During quality-of-life discussions, I often ask my clients, "What does your pet enjoy? What makes them happy?" What is happy for a Border Collie is likely very different from a Basset Hound, but the unifying desire to ensure their comfort and ability to enjoy their life remains constant.

It wasn't until later in my career that I began to ponder the happiness of the humans in the exam room: the client, myself, and my colleagues. What was our quality of life, and shouldn't that be considered as important as our patients? Because truly, at that point in my career, I was suffering. It was also at that point that I began work with a suicide prevention organization called Not One More Vet (NOMV). My work there has exposed me to the breadth of what concerns us as a profession, introduced me to amazing experts in social work and psychology, and deepened my understanding of how we can all care for ourselves with as much enthusiasm as we show for our patients. It has also opened the eyes to the discomfort of not just my veterinarian colleagues but also the support team members who work alongside us. Much of the literature up to this point has focused on the veterinarian; however, all of the human beings we work with deserve a good quality of life. Moreover, a growing body of knowledge suggests that the well-being of veterinary support staff has similar, if not greater, challenges than that of the veterinarians they work with (Witte et al. 2019; Kramper et al. 2023; Volk

et al. 2024). The term "veterinary professionals" is used in this text with the intention to identify all people who work in the veterinary field, and data regarding support staff well-being will be included whenever possible. The well-being of the profession as a whole depends on all of its members, not just those with a doctorate.

My pursuit of happiness took the same methodology as my career, seeking a scientific basis for practices and applying them in a practical way. This book reflects that methodology. We will cover the empirical literature on the topic presented, and also provide stories from veterinary professionals across the globe. Through this exploration, we will cover the breadth of both what challenges our quality of life and also how we can both protect and enhance that well-being. The end goal of this book is to help you, the veterinary professional, understand and ultimately find your own happiness, and to value it as you do the well-being of your patients.

WHAT IS HAPPINESS?

> *[Happiness is] the experience of joy, contentment, or positive wellbeing, combined with a sense that one's life is good, meaningful, and worthwhile.*
>
> Sonja Lyubomirsky 2007

As familiar as the term "happiness" is, an encompassing, universally accepted definition can be difficult to pin down. It has been debated by ancient philosophers, continuing into modern day. At its most basic level, happiness is related to pleasure. Hedonism is happiness related to a pleasurable sensory experience. Something tastes good, looks beautiful, sounds nice, etc. If this were all that happiness entailed, then our goal would simply be to maximize those pleasures in life. However, when polled, people don't actually aspire to continually maximizing pleasure. On average, people aspire to experience pleasure between 70% and 80% of their lives (Hornsey et al. 2018).

From this research, it is apparent that people expect some negative experiences. Arguably, we will even seek it out. For example, careers in veterinary medicine, which involve numerous stressors, are not entirely pleasant. However, many people, including people reading this textbook, go to great lengths to work in this field. And why is that? This field also brings a sense of purpose and meaning to life, which encompasses a different type of happiness called eudaimonia. This type of happiness was first defined by Aristotle, who outlined that eudaimonia was not only desirable but the entire aim of human existence (Egbekpalu 2021). True to Aristotle's assertions, when studied, a sense of meaning and purpose was determined to be a key aspect of happiness in veterinary professionals (Cake et al. 2015).

The dichotomy of hedonism and eudaimonia brings us to a more nuanced view of happiness, called subjective well-being. Subjective well-being is defined as the way an individual perceives and experiences their life, and it measures both the emotional or hedonistic aspects, as well as the cognitive or eudaimonic aspects of happiness. Quality-of-life researcher and professor of psychology Robert A. Cummins also asserted the concept of balance or a sense of homeostasis in mood as an important concept in well-being (David et al. 2014). Ultimately, the goal of this book is to help the reader achieve a healthy emotional homeostasis, where negative experiences are processed quickly, so that the individual can return to a baseline and fully appreciate the pleasures in life when they happen.

ARE VETERINARY PROFESSIONALS HAPPY?

Much like the definition of happiness, the answer to the question "Are veterinary professionals happy?" is a complicated one. As will be discussed at length in this text, there are troubling statistics like elevated psychological distress, suicide rates, and burnout among veterinary professionals (Nett et al. 2015; Ouedraogo et al. 2021; Witte et al. 2019). A majority of veterinarians report facing distressing situations on a daily basis (Kipperman et al. 2017). There are numerous studies on veterinary well-being, and a majority of them focus on the negative well-being metrics such as stress, suicide, anxiety, and depression (Cake et al. 2017).

Certainly, well-being concerns exist within the field, but they do not present the full story. When polled, 80% of veterinarians report being satisfied, very satisfied, or extremely satisfied with their jobs (Ashton-James and McNeilage 2022). Furthermore, more than three-quarters of veterinarians would consider veterinary medicine as a career path if given the chance to start over again (Robinson et al. 2019). Many veterinary professionals are not just professionally satisfied, but emotionally happy as well. More than half the veterinarians in a 2019 survey reported feeling good about themselves and cheerful often or all of the time, and 85% felt that way at least some of the time (Robinson et al. 2019). Clearly, there is a great deal of happiness to be found in our field.

WHAT DETERMINES OUR HAPPINESS?

In her foundational work, positive psychologist Sonya Lyubomirsky categorized three areas that determine our happiness: genetics, circumstances, and positive activity. Figure 1.1 shows the relative contribution of each of these aspects to our general happiness (Lyubomirsky et al. 2005).

The largest component of happiness is genetic in origin. In a study of long-term well-being, identical twins had a substantial concordance in their scores (40%), where fraternal twins did not (7%). The concordance was consistent even when the twins were raised in different homes, indicating a strong genetic component to well-being (Lykken and Tellegen 1996). Other studies have shown that other characteristics that have been linked to happiness, such as personality traits, are also at least partially genetic (Zwir et al. 2020). This genetic basis for happiness presents an argument that a good deal of our happiness is out of our control, that we do indeed have an innate happiness set point. Thankfully, this is not the full story.

Although it may seem counterintuitive, our current circumstances (e.g. our relationship status, income, and even our physical health) only impact our happiness by approximately 10% (Lyubomirsky 2007). This impact, however, is not entirely straightforward. For instance, income has a complicated relationship with mental health and happiness. In cross-sectional studies, income has a consistently positive relationship with happiness. This might lead you to think, "If I want to be happier, I need to try to earn more and more money." However, when evaluated over a period of time, increasing income does not increase happiness (Khalil 2022). This

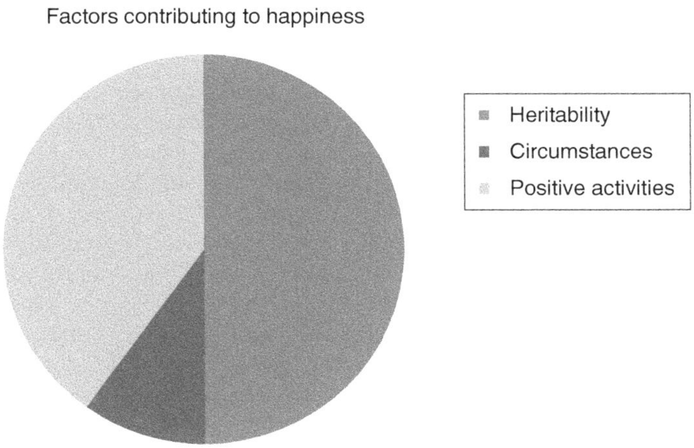

FIGURE 1.1 Happiness chart. Adapted From Lyubomirsky (2005)

paradox seems to be rooted in the varying definitions of happiness. In an oft-quoted study, happiness increased with income up to an annual salary of $75,000, after which happiness and income were not related (Kahneman and Deaton 2010). It is important to distinguish that emotional well-being, or hedonistic happiness, is the type of happiness with a ceiling effect in regard to income. The ceiling effect on hedonistic happiness was related directly to the impact of stressors, where poverty severely exacerbates the emotional impacts of things like health issues, divorce, or other common misfortunes (Kahneman and Deaton 2010). Perhaps money cannot buy happiness, but it seems you can pay your way out of a good deal of unhappiness. For instance, let's say your car, your sole mode of transportation to work, breaks down. If you have the resources to get it fixed or replaced, this is a temporary inconvenience in your life. However, if you do not have those resources, this represents a significant impact on your life, leading to numerous other stressors. You can't get to work, which means you can't make money, which means you can't afford your other bills, etc. Once an income level has been achieved where those stressors can be handled without undue hardship, the impact of income on emotional well-being becomes negligible.

The impact of circumstantial change on happiness also has a tendency to be temporary due to a phenomenon called hedonistic adaptation, where people tend to return to a relatively stable level of happiness over time (Sheldon and Lyubomirsky 2021). For instance, in a longitudinal study of relationships, there is an initial boost in emotional well-being in the months leading up to marriage, but after marriage, this either stabilizes or declines (Huntington et al. 2022). There are two factors that contribute to this adaptation. The first is habituation to the new circumstances. When a change is new, it presents a variety of novel, positive experiences, which in turn result in positive emotions. As the novelty wears off, so does the experience of the positive emotions.

The second is a matter of perspective. As the positive experiences become the new norm, adaptation occurs, and aspirations tend to shift to a higher level of expectations (Sheldon and Lyubomirsky 2021). This presents a never-ending treadmill of expectations, requiring even more positive events to gain the same level of satisfaction, which unfortunately can cause a decline in well-being (Sheldon and Lyubomirsky 2021). In Story 1.1, a veterinarian describes how this shift in expectations impacted her in vet school. In this example, we see that what should have been a source of pride and accomplishment becomes a source of stress, as a new, harder goal is

STORY 1.1 THE HEDONISTIC TREADMILL

When I entered vet school, I knew that I wanted to specialize. I also knew that meant I needed to focus on my grades. To give myself the best chance at a competitive residency, I set a goal of being in the top 10% of my class. Needless to say, vet school was harder than my wildest dreams. The amount of effort I used to put in for As and Bs just wasn't cutting it. So I really stepped up my game, and it paid off. At the end of the first semester, I checked my class rank and found out that I was, in fact, the top student in my class. I was so proud of myself, so excited. This achievement made me reach for an even higher goal where nothing but being the top student in the class would do. I spent the next four years torturing myself over every grade, every assignment, so I wouldn't lose that top spot. I studied ridiculous hours. I didn't have a social life. I missed family events all in pursuit of this goal. Despite all of that struggle, at the end of it all, I graduated second in my class due to a snowstorm that kept me from an exam. It's absurd to me that I can sit here now as a specialist, having achieved everything that I wanted, and still feel frustrated—disappointed even—about my class rank because I didn't reach the even more ridiculous goal I had set for myself.

substituted with no real justification. The well-being impacts of that moved goal post are seen long-term, as the doctor still feels frustrated about an objectively excellent performance in veterinary school, despite the achievement of her original goal of becoming a specialist.

The relationship between happiness and circumstances does seem to be more complex when viewed through the lens of life satisfaction. It is interesting to note that in Kahneman and Deaton (2010) study, when a more eudaimonic measure was used, logarithmic income and happiness had a positive, linear relationship across income brackets (Kahneman and Deaton 2010). As another example, marriage is weakly associated with long-term life satisfaction. However, that effect is significantly mediated by other factors, such as beliefs toward marriage. People who believe in the importance of marriage and who are married report higher life satisfaction (Moss and Willoughby 2018). Once again, it seems that expectations have an important role to play when determining how circumstances impact well-being. However, the impact of that belief on life satisfaction was further moderated by other factors like age, gender, education level, and religion, sometimes turning the association into a negative one. A single life circumstance may be associated on the whole with life satisfaction; however, a multitude of other factors can change or even negate its impact.

Given that we cannot change our genetics and that circumstantial changes have only a partial, perhaps temporary impact, you may conclude that there is a happiness set point that cannot be significantly altered. Thankfully, a number of techniques have been shown in peer review to increase our overall well-being, contributing to approximately 40% of our happiness (Lyubomirsky et al. 2005). Chapter 10 will focus specifically on these techniques. The rest of this chapter will focus on the overall concept and methodology of improving well-being through positive activity.

Some authors have since challenged the extent of the impact that positive activities can have, disputing Lyubomirsky's original estimate of 40%. Lyubomirsky herself has said that, since the original publication, the effect of positive activities may have been overstated in her original model (Lyubomirsky et al. 2011). In fact, over the years, a great deal of variance in the impact of positive interventions has been found, ranging from 8% to 65% (White et al. 2019). Regardless of the exact figure, research continues to show a significant impact of positive activities on our well-being (Carr et al. 2021; Klug and Maier 2015). Story 1.2 demonstrates how a wellness intervention had a positive impact on one veterinarian's ability to handle a problem at her practice.

STORY 1.2 THREE GOOD THINGS

I am a naturally neurotic and fairly pessimistic person. My therapist actually explained that these can be helpful traits as a doctor. Do you think about how things might go wrong and the 15 different plans you have on how to react? You can be my surgeon any day. Quickly recognizing problems and risks, and considering potential negative outcomes, is an important skill in medicine.

But at some point, all of the negative spirals in my brain were doing a number on my mental health. After reading a bit about the impacts of gratitude exercises, I started doing the Three Good Things exercise. In this exercise, you write down three specific and small things you are grateful for in the last 24 hours. Things like "I had a good hair day" or "That client was really nice." I did this twice a week for a couple of years, basically training my brain to look for bright spots.

And late one night, I had the perfect experience of how that exercise has helped me. I had just sat on my couch after a very long day when I got a text from our custodian, Mario. My brand-new practice, which I finished construction on less than two months prior, had a leak. In fact, there was water pouring out of the electrical outlets.

STORY 1.2 (CONTINUED)

Previously, news like this would have sent me into a full-blown pity party. I would have grumbled about it all night, and likely well into the following week. However, after the work I had done on gratitude exercises, I had a very different experience.

I jump in my car to run back over to the practice and think to myself, "thank god I charged my car last night, otherwise I wouldn't have the juice to get there." I arrive and Mario shows me the leak, and I think to myself, "Mario is a really great custodian who really goes above and beyond. I'm so thankful he saw it and caught some video." I get the big ladder out and am momentarily grateful that the contractors left this huge ladder at the practice, even though I was a bit annoyed about it clogging up the storage room last week. I crawl up on the roof above that room and see the problem. Our Heating Ventilation and Air Conditioning (HVAC) system has overflowed its condensation tray. Said tray is supposed to have a drain, which is clearly not working. I text my contractor. He replies: "Yeah, the HVAC guy said he had a concern last week." Am I a bit miffed that I'm hearing about this now that it is an emergency? You betcha. The contractor assures me that someone will be there in the morning. So I'm annoyed, but satisfied that a long-term solution is in motion. For tonight, I just need a temporary fix. I haul the shop vac I bought two weeks ago up the ladder. As I am doing so, I note that it is now approaching 9 pm, and I think to myself, "Thank God I bought this shop vac for the fish tank, and I'm not rushing to the Home Depot before it closes."

Was I thrilled to drive back to work after a long day? Absolutely not. Am I happy that my contractor neglected to handle this before it became a problem? Absolutely not. But I'm not furious. I'm not crying. I'm not obsessing about what else might go wrong. Every one of those tiny bright spots pulled me back from the doom spiral my brain would have fallen into before I started gratitude practices, and for that I am grateful. I dealt with the problem and got back to baseline pretty quickly. By the time I sat back down on the couch an hour later, I was ready to enjoy the rest of the evening. That's a big change for my ability to emotionally process problems.

THE PATH TO HAPPINESS

Becoming happier takes both a will and a proper way.

Sonya Lyubomirsky et al. 2011

Unfortunately, the path to happiness is not always an easy one. The first hurdle we face is one of motivation. In a 2010 study, two ads were placed for participants in a study. The first ad called for people who wanted to increase their happiness, the second asked for participants for a study on cognitive exercises, thereby sorting participants into those motivated to improve their happiness vs those without that explicit motivation (Lyubomirsky et al. 2011). All participants were then randomly assigned to one of two experimental conditions: either optimism or gratitude exercises, or the control condition, which involved journaling about last week's activities. Several interesting observations came from this study. First, all motivated participants assigned to either experimental condition had an increase in well-being both at eight weeks and six months, and those assigned to the control condition did not. This combats the idea that motivation alone is enough. You cannot just simply "choose happiness" and have it appear.

However, motivation should not be completely discounted. Motivated participants in the experimental group had greater gains in well-being in both the short- and long-term compared to unmotivated participants and controls. Furthermore, the amount of effort that participants put into the exercises was directly related to increases in well-being. So from this study, we see that we must have both the will and the way to improve our own well-being. The interventions can have positive impacts, but those impacts are moderated by both our motivation and the effort we put toward them.

The remainder of this text explores the many factors that may impact our well-being and provides a framework and tools to improve your own quality of life. The motivation to improve and the efforts therein, however, are up to you. I do hope that this text provides you with a grounded view of well-being and a belief that you can do better for yourself and your colleagues. With motivation and effort, I know we can have positive impacts on the lives of not only our patients but also ourselves.

REFERENCES

Ashton-James, C.E. and McNeilage, A.G. (2022). A mixed methods investigation of stress and wellbeing factors contributing to burnout and job satisfaction in a specialist small animal hospital. *Frontiers in Veterinary Science* 9: 942778.

Cake, M.A., Bell, M.A., Bickley, N., and Bartram, D.J. (2015). The life of meaning: a model of the positive contributions to well-being from veterinary work. *Journal of Veterinary Medical Education* 42 (3): 184–193.

Cake, M.A., McArthur, M.M., Matthew, S.M., and Mansfield, C.F. (2017). Finding the balance: uncovering resilience in the veterinary literature. *Journal of Veterinary Medical Education* 44 (1): 95–105.

Carr, A., Cullen, K., Keeney, C. et al. (2021). Effectiveness of positive psychology interventions: a systematic review and meta-analysis. *The Journal of Positive Psychology* 16 (6): 749–769.

David, S.A., Boniwell, I., and Ayers, A.C. (ed.) (2014). *The Oxford handbook of happiness*. Oxford University Press.

Egbekpalu, P.E. (2021). Aristotelian concept of happiness (eudaimonia) and its conative role in human existence: A critical evaluation. *Conatus-Journal of Philosophy* 6 (2): 75–86.

Hornsey, M.J., Bain, P.G., Harris, E.A. et al. (2018). How much is enough in a perfect world? Cultural variation in ideal levels of happiness, pleasure, freedom, health, self-esteem, longevity, and intelligence. *Psychological Science* 29 (9): 1393–1404.

Huntington, C., Stanley, S.M., Doss, B.D., and Rhoades, G.K. (2022). Happy, healthy, and wedded? How the transition to marriage affects mental and physical health. *Journal of Family Psychology* 36 (4): 608.

Kahneman, D. and Deaton, A. (2010). High income improves evaluation of life but not emotional well-being. *Proceedings of the National Academy of Sciences* 107 (38): 16489–16493.

Khalil, E.L. (2022). Solving the income-happiness paradox. *International Review of Economics* 69 (3): 433–463.

Kipperman, B.S., Kass, P.H., and Rishniw, M. (2017). Factors that influence small animal veterinarians' opinions and actions regarding cost of care and effects of economic limitations on patient care and outcome and professional career satisfaction and burnout. *Journal of the American Veterinary Medical Association* 250 (7): 785–794.

Klug, H.J. and Maier, G.W. (2015). Linking goal progress and subjective well-being: A meta-analysis. *Journal of Happiness Studies* 16: 37–65.

Kramper, S., Crosby, E.S., Waitz-Kudla, S.N. et al. (2023). Highly stressful events and posttraumatic stress disorder symptoms among veterinary professionals: Prevalence and associations with mental health and job-related outcomes. *Psychological Trauma Theory Research Practice and Policy* 15 (Suppl 2): S275–S285. https://doi.org/10.1037/tra0001432.

Lykken, D. and Tellegen, A. (1996). Happiness is a stochastic phenomenon. *Psychological Science* 7 (3): 186–189.

Lyubomirsky, S. (2007). *The How of Happiness: A New Approach to Getting the Life You Want*, 37. New York, USA: Penguin Press.

Lyubomirsky, S., Dickerhoof, R., Boehm, J.K., and Sheldon, K.M. (2011). Becoming happier takes both a will and a proper way: an experimental longitudinal intervention to boost well-being. *Emotion* 11 (2): 391.

Lyubomirsky, S., Sheldon, K.M., and Schkade, D. (2005). Pursuing happiness: the architecture of sustainable change. *Review of General Psychology* 9: 111–131.

Moss, E. and Willoughby, B.J. (2018). Associations between beliefs about marriage and life satisfaction: the moderating role of relationship status and gender. *Journal of Family Studies* 24 (3): 274–290.

Nett, R.J., Witte, T.K., Holzbauer, S.M. et al. (2015). Risk factors for suicide, attitudes toward mental illness, and practice-related stressors among US veterinarians. *Journal of the American Veterinary Medical Association* 247 (8): 945–955.

Ouedraogo, F.B., Lefebvre, S.L., Hansen, C.R., and Brorsen, B.W. (2021). Compassion satisfaction, burnout, and secondary traumatic stress among full-time veterinarians in the United States (2016–2018). *Journal of the American Veterinary Medical Association* 258 (11): 1259–1270.

Robinson, D., Edwards, M., Mason, B. et al. (2019). *The 2019 Survey of the Veterinary Profession*. Brighton, UK: Institute for Employment Studies.

Sheldon, K.M. and Lyubomirsky, S. (2021). Revisiting the sustainable happiness model and pie chart: Can happiness be successfully pursued? *The Journal of Positive Psychology* 16 (2): 145–154.

Volk, J.O., Schimmack, U., Strand, E.B. et al. (2024). Merck Animal Health Veterinary Team study reveals factors associated with well-being, burnout, and mental health among nonveterinarian practice team members. *Journal of the American Veterinary Medical Association* 1 (aop): 1–5.

White, C.A., Uttl, B., and Holder, M.D. (2019). Meta-analyses of positive psychology interventions: the effects are much smaller than previously reported. *PLoS One* 14 (5): e0216588.

Witte, T.K., Spitzer, E.G., Edwards, N. et al. (2019). Suicides and deaths of undetermined intent among veterinary professionals from 2003 through 2014. *Journal of the American Veterinary Medical Association* 255 (5): 595–608.

Zwir, I., Arnedo, J., Del-Val, C. et al. (2020). Uncovering the complex genetics of human character. *Molecular Psychiatry* 25 (10): 2295–2312.

The Individual and Well-Being CHAPTER 2

Carrie Jurney, DVM, DACVIM (Neurology)[1] and Jesse S. Michel, PhD[2]

[1] *Not One More Vet, Inc, San Francisco, CA, USA*

[2] *Department of Psychological Sciences, Auburn University, Auburn, AL, USA*

INTRODUCTION

As we set the stage for discussing well-being in veterinary medicine, two domains deserve particular attention: who veterinary professionals are as people and the working environments we share. When examining the well-being challenges of a profession, it is tempting to focus solely on structural or occupational factors. Yet personality plays a substantial role in shaping how individuals perceive, respond to, and recover from workplace stress. In fact, a study examining the relative contributions of workplace stressors and personality traits found that personality accounted for more variance in occupational stress among veterinarians than work factors alone (Dawson & Thompson 2017). This perspective is echoed in qualitative research, in which approximately half of the interviewed veterinarians, unprompted, described their personality traits as factors they believed predisposed them to stress or difficulty (Platt et al. 2012).

Based on this research, one can imagine a scenario in which two veterinarians are working at the same clinic. They have the same schedule, the same case complexity, the same staffing ratios, and yet one of these clinicians is crying in the bathroom from stress, while the other is sailing through the day, cracking jokes with their team. What's the difference? Their baseline personality, along with the coping mechanisms and personal resources they have cultivated, allows them to process stressors differently, changing their emotional impact. Perhaps the doctor who is laughing with the team has a lower baseline level of neuroticism, which has allowed them have a more positive mindset. Indeed, a 2016 study showed that a person's level of neuroticism accounts for 16% of the variance in the emotional impact of stressors in the moment in part because neuroticism makes those stressors seem more severe and less controllable (Leger et al. 2016). Perhaps the less impacted doctor is also high in conscientiousness, a trait characterized by orderliness, self-control, and deliberate planning. Conscientiousness appears to buffer stress reactivity by reducing both the number and severity of perceived stressors (Leger et al. 2016). It's also possible that the two doctors have very similar baseline personalities, but the less impacted doctor has been practicing mindfulness, which is helping them process stress in this moment. Mindfulness and other positive psychology exercises will be discussed in Chapter 10. Taken together, this example shows that while our environment sets the stage for stress, individual personality differences and learned coping skills largely determine how those stressors are interpreted and felt.

In this chapter, we will explore the aspects of our personalities that can predispose us to and shield us from stressors and the subsequent impacts on our well-being.

PERSONALITY THEORY

Over the years, researchers have developed a range of models to explain personality. Scientifically validated frameworks increasingly view personality as a set of traits that exist along a spectrum, rather than assigning individuals to fixed categories.

Table 2.1 The Big Five personality traits.

Trait	Description	Example characteristics
Openness to experience	Reflects curiosity, imagination, and preference for novelty and variety. People high in openness are often creative, intellectually curious, and open to new experiences.	Imaginative, curious, original, artistic, insightful
Conscientiousness	Describes self-discipline, organization, and goal-directed behavior. High scorers tend to be reliable and deliberate; low scorers are more spontaneous and flexible.	Organized, dependable, disciplined, thorough, responsible
Extraversion	Captures sociability, assertiveness, and positive emotionality. High scorers seek stimulation and social interaction.	Outgoing, energetic, talkative, enthusiastic, sociable
Agreeableness	Reflects interpersonal orientation, compassion, and cooperation versus antagonism and suspicion.	Kind, trusting, altruistic, sympathetic, cooperative
Neuroticism	Indicates emotional instability and tendency toward negative emotions such as anxiety and moodiness.	Anxious, tense, self-conscious, vulnerable, moody

Sources: Costa and McCrae (1992), Goldberg (1990).

One of the earlier biologically informed personality theories is Eysenck's (1967) Psychoticism Extraversion Neuroticism (PEN) model, which connects nervous system functioning and hormonal influences to three core traits: psychoticism (impulsivity and antisocial tendencies), extraversion (sociability and stimulation-seeking), and neuroticism (emotional instability). Another is Cattell and Mead's (2008) 16 Personality Factors model, which distinguishes between observable surface traits and deeper source traits and emphasizes the influence of context and environment on personality expression. Building on these earlier theories, the Five-Factor Model (FFM), popularized by Costa and McCrae (1992) and supported by researchers like Goldberg, has become a pervasive framework in personality research. The FFM proposes five broad, higher-order traits: openness, conscientiousness, extraversion, agreeableness, and neuroticism (see Table 2.1).

The Big Five personality traits capture the major clustering patterns of personality traits. Still, the idea that there are precisely five broad traits is not sacrosanct. In psychology, long-running debates about whether behavior is driven more by personality or by the situation have largely settled on a middle ground: traits and situations jointly shape behavior (Li 2023). Cross-cultural research shows that the Big Five framework works well in general, although different cultures can show variations (Mezquita et al. 2019; Rolland 2002). Modern statistical methods support these findings but also show that other models, such as Zuckerman's psychobiological five, can fit certain datasets (Rossier et al. 2007). In practical terms, trait scores should be understood as tendencies rather than strict predictions. They are influenced by context, and they make the most sense when interpreted alongside real-world situations and an individual's values (Boyle et al. 2008; Kuper et al. 2021).

In contrast to trait models, type-based models assign individuals to rigid personality categories. Popular examples include the Enneagram, Myers–Briggs Type Indicator (MBTI), and the DISC model (Radisavljević et al. 2023; Osborn et al. 2024). These schemas are often used in corporate settings for team building or personnel selection (Rinjani, 2023). While appealing for their simplicity and approachability, these tools have significant limitations. Research shows that type-based models suffer from poor test–retest reliability – people often receive different results upon retesting – and low predictive validity in workplace or behavioral outcomes (Pittenger 1993; Capraro and Capraro 2002; Hook et al. 2021). Critics also argue that these instruments oversimplify personality by forcing complex individual differences into fixed categories. While they may offer some insights in informal or team-building contexts, they lack the scientific rigor needed for research and critical decision-making. They will therefore not be discussed further in this chapter.

THE BIG FIVE AND WELL-BEING

The Big Five personality traits are widely recognized as predictors of well-being outcomes both broadly and specifically within veterinary medicine (Dawson and Thompson 2017; Strickhouser et al. 2017). For example, a meta-analysis of more than 500,000 participants showed that the Big Five personality traits are reliably related to mental health outcomes, with neuroticism showing the most substantial adverse effect ($r = -0.27$; Strickhouser 2017). At the same time, conscientiousness and agreeableness had moderate positive effects ($r = 0.22$ and 0.21, respectively), while extraversion and openness showed modest positive effects ($r = 0.11$ and 0.06, respectively; Strickhouser 2017). Similarly, research has identified neuroticism as a key risk factor for the experience of occupational stress and well-being issues in veterinary professionals (Dawson and Thompson 2017; Volk et al. 2023). Moreover, veterinarians with higher conscientiousness are more likely to engage in proactive mental health behaviors and have fewer burnout symptoms (Dawson and Thompson 2017; Volk et al. 2023).

The consistency of these findings across general and veterinary populations is not surprising. After all, veterinary professionals are human beings, and it stands to reason that the larger trends in personality and well-being would apply. However, the relative levels of various personality traits within the veterinary population offer interesting insights into the interplay between personality and well-being concerns in the field. In longitudinal research, veterinary professionals have shown increases in neuroticism, decreases in extraversion, increases in openness to experience, and relative stability in conscientiousness; support staff show similar trends but have higher neuroticism than veterinarians (Volk et al. 2019, 2021, 2023). These findings, particularly around neuroticism, have further associations with other traits like perfectionism and resilience, which will be explored in the next section.

Given the impact of neuroticism and, to a lesser extent, extraversion, on mental health and well-being in the literature, targeted evaluation and strategic coping mechanisms around these aspects of personality may yield a significant impact on veterinary well-being.

OTHER TRAITS AND WELL-BEING

While the FFM is a robust, validated way to look at personality, it does not necessarily encompass the breadth and depth of all aspects of personality. Certain characteristics, such as empathy and sensory-processing sensitivity (SPS), extend beyond static personality traits and intersect with learned skills and contextual factors. These elements are explored in more depth in the following section. Other phenomena, such as compassion fatigue, burnout, etc., are outcomes rather than traits and are discussed as consequences of sustained empathic labor and poor recovery. These concepts are discussed in Chapters 6 and 7.

Some attributes, like empathy, are not only dispositional but also can be developed through education and experience. Although many of these features correlate with traits in the FFM (e.g. empathy with agreeableness or SPS with neuroticism), they present unique challenges and implications for well-being and professional functioning that warrant separate consideration (Melchers et al. 2016; Colombo et al. 2017; Menor-Campos et al. 2019). For a summary of trait-informed risks, assets, and micro-interventions, see Table 2.2.

EMPATHY

Empathy is defined as the ability to both understand (cognitive empathy) and resonate with (affective empathy) others' emotions. It is widely regarded both as a trainable skill and a personality trait that most strongly correlates with agreeableness, with more modest associations with openness to experience and extraversion (Melchers et al. 2016; Colombo et al. 2017; Guilera et al. 2019). Importantly, empathy is a foundational skill in health care. In human medicine,

Table 2.2 Trait-informed risks, assets, mechanisms, and micro-interventions (veterinary practice).

Trait/construct	Key assets in veterinary practice	Common risks (when unmanaged)	Mechanisms & high-yield micro-interventions
Neuroticism	Vigilance, error-checking. preparedness in high-stakes cases	Threat vigilance → rumination, moral stress reactivity, anxiety/ burnout risk	Mechanisms: negative affect, impaired recovery (low detachment/relaxation). Micro-interventions: brief detachment breaks, relaxation bouts, mindfulness, structured peer debriefs, post-euthanasia recovery protocols.
Conscientiousness	Reliability, adherence to protocols, thoroughness, follow-through	Rigidity, overcontrol, workaholism, perfectionistic concerns	Mechanisms: goal over-persistence, cognitive narrowing. Micro-interventions: timeboxing, "good-enough" checklists, self-compassion prompts, bounded goal-setting, protected time off.
Extraversion	Client communication, team energy, alliance building	Overcommitment to client-facing tasks, overstimulation in noisy/ chaotic settings	Mechanisms: stimulation-seeking, emotional labor. Micro-interventions: balanced scheduling (mix of client and non-client tasks), micro-recovery between consults, noise management.
Agreeableness	Empathy, collaboration, therapeutic alliance, conflict de-escalation	Difficulty setting limits, compassion overextension, decision avoidance	Mechanisms: empathic load, boundary slippage. Micro-interventions: boundary-setting scripts, assertiveness micro-skills, triage/handoff protocols, team norms for saying no.
Openness to experience	Cognitive flexibility, innovation, reflective case formulation, learning orientation	Distraction/scope drift, preference for novelty over protocol	Mechanisms: exploratory attention. Micro-interventions: pre-commit checklists, "idea parking lot," structured reflection, protocol review windows.
Empathy (trait and skill)	Client/practitioner rapport, adherence support, meaning/purpose	Compassion fatigue, emotional exhaustion, moral distress if boundaries weak	Mechanisms: sustained empathic labor, high affective load. Micro-interventions: communication training, peer support, boundary scripts, scheduled recovery, reflective practice.
Perfectionism (adaptive/ maladaptive)	Precision, diligence, high standards when flexible and self-compassionate	Moral stressor sensitivity, concern over mistakes, impaired recovery	Mechanisms: overcontrol, reduced detachment/relaxation. Micro-interventions: self-compassion drills, "done-vs-perfect" rules, after-action reviews focused on learning, protected detachment windows.
Resilience (resource)	Faster recovery, coping repertoire, sustained functioning under strain	Low resilience → susceptibility to distress, withdrawal, burnout	Mechanisms: self-efficacy, coping style, social support. Micro-interventions: coping-skills training, reflective practice, peer/ supervisor support, job-crafting to align strengths.

Table 2.2 (Continued)

Trait/construct	Key assets in veterinary practice	Common risks (when unmanaged)	Mechanisms & high-yield micro-interventions
Sensory-processing sensitivity (SPS)	Fine-grained attunement to animals/clients, recognition of subtle cues	Overstimulation, social stress, emotional fatigue in high-noise/pressure contexts	Mechanisms: heightened sensory/emotional reactivity. Micro-interventions: quiet spaces, noise control, predictable scheduling, boundary-setting, mindfulness, task-mix emphasizing strengths.
Workaholism (pattern)	Short-term productivity, mastery signals	Chronic overwork → burnout, detachment from non-work roles, health risks	Mechanisms: cultural norms + individual overcommitment, recovery deficits. Micro-interventions: explicit hours boundaries, minimum time-off norms, caseload caps, leadership modeling recovery, "no after-hours charting" policies.
Values/person–environment fit	Meaning, retention, ethical coherence	Moral stress under value misfit, disengagement, turnover	Mechanisms: value incongruence amplifies stress. Micro-interventions: explicit value signposting in hiring/onboarding, role design aligned to values, team rituals reinforcing norms.

Translating Evidence into Practice

Table 2.2 Integrates the chapter's findings into a pragmatic map for clinicians and leaders: for each trait or adjacent construct, it summarizes typical assets, unmanaged risks, the mechanisms most often implicated in strain or flourishing, and high-yield micro-interventions that can be built into supervision, scheduling, and team routines. The patterning reflects (a) robust meta-analytic links between the Big Five and mental health (e.g. strongest adverse association for neuroticism; modest protective roles for conscientiousness and agreeableness), (b) veterinary-specific survey evidence on trait levels and well-being correlates, and (c) recovery science emphasizing psychological detachment and relaxation as core pathways for preventing burnout (Sonnentag and Fritz 2015; Dawson and Thompson 2017; Strickhouser et al. 2017). Use the table with, not instead of, contextual assessment (values/person–environment fit, workload, and role clarity) and the plasticity lens developed earlier in this chapter.

Note: Assets and risks represent typical patterns and are context-dependent. Interpret in conjunction with the chapter sections on the Big Five, other traits, and plasticity. Key sources: Big Five & well-being effects (Dawson and Thompson 2017; Strickhouser et al. 2017); recovery mechanisms and detachment/relaxation (Sonnentag and Fritz 2015); mindfulness buffering of neuroticism (Giluk 2009); perfectionism in veterinary contexts (Stoeber and Childs 2011; Crane et al. 2015; Holden 2020); empathy outcomes and training (Derksen et al. 2013; Pizzolon et al. 2019; Winter et al. 2020; Varela and Correia 2023); resilience determinants/interventions (Cake et al. 2017; Perret et al. 2020; McArthur et al. 2021); SPS correlates and implications (Listou Grimen and Diseth 2016; Pérez-Chacón et al. 2021; Morellini et al. 2023); workaholism and organizational levers (Lakkawar et al. 2020; Steffey et al. 2023); and values/P–E fit and moral stress (Cake et al. 2015).

provider empathy has been robustly linked to greater patient satisfaction, improved adherence to treatment plans, and better overall health outcomes (Derksen et al. 2013). Echoing this, empathetic client communications were related to both increases in following treatment recommendations and, in turn, client satisfaction (Kanji et al. 2012).

Empathy levels vary across both demographic and professional factors. Female veterinary professionals and students tend to have higher empathy scores than male veterinary professionals and students (Colombo et al. 2017; Menor-Campos et al. 2019). This is consistent with broader psychological research indicating that women generally score higher on empathy, likely reflecting sociocultural and psychosocial influences (Menor-Campos et al. 2019). Veterinary support staff often report even higher levels of affective empathy than veterinarians, a pattern attributed to their frequent, direct contact with both patients and clients (Pizzolon et al. 2019; Varela and Correia 2023).

Empathy also changes with experience. Students who have previously worked with animal welfare organizations demonstrate higher empathy, highlighting the influence of experience and environment on empathic development (Menor-Campos et al. 2019). Importantly, in veterinary medicine, empathy has two targets: the patient and the client. The split, and at times conflicting, nature of veterinary empathy can contribute to stressful moments. Empathy for a patient's suffering can quickly morph into frustration with a client who cannot afford treatment. The relative levels of empathy to these targets also evolve over the course of a career, with more experienced clinicians showing higher levels of client-directed empathy (Colombo et al. 2017).

While central to job performance, empathy has a complicated relationship to well-being. Empathy strengthens client relationships and even patient outcomes, but it can also increase the risk of burnout, compassion fatigue, and moral distress, particularly when emotional boundaries are not well maintained (Varela and Correia 2023). Among veterinarians, higher empathy scores have been associated with both greater professional fulfillment and an increased susceptibility to emotional exhaustion, highlighting empathy's dual role as both a resource and a risk (Pizzolon et al. 2019; Varela and Correia 2023).

These effects may be even more pronounced among veterinary support staff, whose frequent direct contact with clients and animals often demands sustained emotional labor and exposes them to distressing experiences (Pizzolon et al. 2019). In turn, compassion fatigue and burnout can diminish empathy capacity through emotional exhaustion, stripping clinicians and staff of this vital skill (Wilkinson et al. 2017). However, empathy also remains a key source of meaning and professional satisfaction, contributing to the sense of purpose many veterinary professionals find in their work (Cake et al. 2015). Supporting well-being, therefore, requires a balanced approach. Empathy can be nurtured through communication training and role modeling (Winter et al. 2020), while its emotional toll can be mitigated through coping strategies, peer support, and boundary-setting (Varela and Correia 2023).

PERFECTIONISM

Perfectionism is a personality trait characterized by striving for flawlessness and setting high performance standards. Some authors describe perfectionism as a common, even pervasive, trait among veterinarians (Dawson & Thompson 2017; Holden 2020). In more quantitative studies, the level of perfectionism in veterinary students is higher than that of college students, but lower than other professional students (Lewis and Cardwell 2020; Karaffa et al. 2024).

Perfectionism can be self-focused (i.e. expecting perfection from yourself), other-focused (i.e. expecting perfection from others), or socially prescribed (i.e. feeling that others expect perfection from you; Smith et al. 2019). In a large meta-analysis, neuroticism was the trait most strongly correlated with perfectionism. Socially prescribed perfectionism, as well as some aspects of self-focused perfectionism, such as concern about making mistakes and doubts about one's own actions, show the most robust associations with neuroticism (Smith et al. 2019). Similar findings have been reported in veterinary populations, where socially and self-oriented perfectionism are strongly correlated with neuroticism with a large effect size (Holden 2020). On the flip side, conscientiousness has been associated with decreased perfectionism in both general and veterinary populations (Smith et al. 2019; Holden 2020).

Perfectionism isn't an entirely negative trait, and in fact can have some benefits. In research, this dichotomy is referred to as adaptive vs maladaptive perfectionism. Adaptive perfectionism, which combines high personal standards with flexibility and self-compassion, is associated with conscientiousness (Stoeber and Childs 2011). However, maladaptive perfectionism is marked by excessive self-criticism and concern over mistakes and is often linked to neuroticism (Stoeber and Childs 2011).

We see reflections of maladaptive perfectionism's impact in the veterinary literature. For instance, in a survey of the emotional effects of medical errors, 36% of veterinarians who had made an error with no consequences to a patient reported long-term negative impacts on their professional life, including considering a career change (Kogan et al. 2018). If a single mistake without consequences makes over a third of us question a career choice that took years of higher education to achieve, it's fair to say that our personal standards are a bit too high. Perfectionism is also one of the most common presenting concerns for vet students attending counseling sessions (Karaffa et al. 2025). It has been shown to increase the impacts of moral stressors in veterinarians, increasing psychological distress (Crane et al. 2015). In addition, maladaptive perfectionistic traits (e.g. concern over mistakes and overcontrol) are associated with impaired recovery from work, hindering psychological detachment and relaxation–two core recovery experiences robustly linked to burnout risk (Sonnentag and Fritz 2015).

Adaptive perfectionism is less represented in the veterinary well-being literature, which may reflect on overall bias toward studies on negative mental health and well-being outcomes (Cake et al. 2017). Adaptive perfectionism includes qualities like precision, diligence, and accountability, which are certainly desirable in a health care setting (Holden 2020; Stoeber and Childs 2011). Moreover, adaptive perfectionism has been shown to benefit health care workers themselves by increasing self-efficacy (the belief that we can achieve our goals), which, in turn, decreases burnout (Ghanim et al. 2025).

In Story 2.1, this duality is illustrated through the experiences of a hospice veterinarian. Her precision and accountability, particularly in the aftercare of remains, reflect both strong professional standards and deep respect for her clients. Yet even when the same care is applied to the euthanasia procedure itself, clinical medicine remains imperfect. Rare and unpredictable reactions can occur, and perfectionism can amplify their emotional impact. Although this practitioner is highly skilled in euthanasia and reports a 99.9% success rate, a single, extremely rare complication has led to lingering frustration and self-doubt about an otherwise proven protocol.

Addressing maladaptive perfectionism through interventions that promote self-awareness and compassion, realistic goal-setting, boundary-setting, and recovery behaviors (e.g. scheduled detachment and relaxation) may help professionals retain its benefits while mitigating its risks (Ståhlberg 2015; Goswami and Baksi 2025).

STORY 2.1 THE PROS AND CONS OF PERFECTIONISM

I work as a home hospice veterinarian. There are certain parts of my job where my perfectionism is a vital skill. For instance, you only have one chance to get crematory aftercare right. One of the worst things I can do is not go over all of the aftercare, or not answer questions, or worse, partner with an awful crematory I wouldn't trust. We simply cannot change the decisions made- do they want a paw print, for instance after the body has been processed. These are extremely important keepsakes of someone's loved one. You have to get that right.

The hard part is controlling my expectations and frustrations with the process. Even though I have carefully selected protocols and strive to do everything right, complications still happen. For example, I was with a rather nervous family outside in 20-degree freezing cold because that's where their Bernese Mountain Dog was comfortable. She was seven years old and was recently diagnosed with cancer in the liver and spleen. I used my regular protocol that I've used over 6,000 times, and the dog sedated really smoothly. Her breathing was a little rapid, and it was making dad nervous, so I was just soothing and moved on to part two. Gave my euthasol IV into the lateral saphenous, well seated in the vein. Was completely done giving it, dog turned her head, gave a breathy screech, and died. I've only ever had that one other time in my career. It's so incredibly frustrating not to understand why that happened and what I can do to make sure that never happens again.

RESILIENCE

Resilience refers to dynamic processes that enable individuals to sustain or regain psychological functioning in the face of stress. In veterinary practice, resilience is shaped by self-efficacy, coping strategies (e.g. problem-focused vs emotion-focused, discussed in Chapter 10), social and supervisory support, and personal resources (e.g. optimism; Cake et al. 2017; McArthur et al. 2021).

Evidence shows that resilience varies across career stages and is associated with better mental health outcomes in veterinarians (Perret et al. 2020). Personality traits contribute to resilience profiles -- for example, higher conscientiousness and lower neuroticism generally predict stronger resilience -- but the relationship is not deterministic (Eley et al. 2013). Importantly, resilience is trainable: targeted interventions (e.g. coping-skills training, reflective practice, and peer support) and supportive job design can strengthen adaptive responses to stress (Cake et al. 2017; Perret et al. 2020; McArthur et al. 2021; Unjai et al. 2024).

Within veterinary education, perfectionism and neuroticism have been linked to lower resilience, underscoring the importance of coaching on self-compassion, realistic goal-setting, and recovery behaviors (Holden 2020). Embedding resilience skills throughout training and early career transitions may promote well-being and retention.

SENSORY-PROCESSING SENSITIVITY

SPS is a personality trait characterized by deeper cognitive processing of sensory input, heightened emotional reactivity, and increased sensitivity to subtle stimuli (Listou Grimen and Diseth 2016). Individuals high in SPS, often referred to as highly sensitive persons (HSPs), tend to be intuitive, empathetic, and responsive to the moods and needs of others. While not part of the Big Five, SPS tends to correlate positively with neuroticism and openness; associations with extraversion are mixed and context-dependent (Listou Grimen and Diseth 2016).

Research suggests that between 15% and 30% of people show high SPS, implying that SPS is a relatively common trait (Aron and Aron 1997; Pluess et al. 2018). Within veterinary medicine, the prevalence of SPS has not been formally studied. Still, the trait is frequently discussed in relation to strong attunement to animals, heightened empathy, and a preference for meaningful one-on-one interactions, which are characteristics thought to be strengths in animal care roles, where attention to subtle behavioral and emotional cues is key (Aron et al. 2012; Pérez-Chacón et al. 2021; Setti et al. 2022). At the same time, this sensitivity can increase vulnerability to emotional fatigue, overstimulation, and social stress, particularly in fast-paced or noisy environments (Morellini et al. 2023). Anyone who has spent a busy day in a treatment area with a persistently barking dog can appreciate how heightened sensory input may amplify daily stress, even when it also supports high-quality patient care.

Sensitivity to sensory stimuli is also commonly associated with neurodivergent conditions such as autism spectrum disorder (Damatac et al. 2025). Autistic individuals are also described as having a strong connection to animals, which, as discussed, is also seen among those with high SPS (Atherton et al. 2023). Well-known examples can further reinforce this perceived overlap. Dr. Temple Grandin, for instance, has described how her autistic sensory experiences shaped her ability to interpret animal behavior. Taken together, these associations make it easy to assume that SPS is simply another way of describing neurodivergence rather than a distinct personality trait.

Research, however, suggests a more nuanced relationship. When SPS has been examined alongside autistic traits, it shows modest overlap with certain features of autism but is not associated with total levels of autistic traits (Damatac et al. 2025). Some similarities do emerge, particularly under adverse conditions. In stressful environments, individuals with higher SPS and those with higher autistic traits both report increased stress (Damatac et al. 2025). However, SPS does not include some of the broader cognitive or social characteristics associated with autism. For example, neuroimaging studies indicate that autism is associated with reduced activation in brain regions

STORY 2.2 NAVIGATING SENSORY SENSITIVITY

Story A: Coping with Sensory Sensitivities In Practice

I have some sound sensitivities, and I've found that Loop earplugs help me filter out some of the background noise in the clinic. I'm also probably more generous with "hospitality" meds than some of my other cohort. I kind of assume that if they're barking enough to be annoying to me, it's probably annoying for them to be that anxious, and they deserve some gabapentin/trazodone.

I absolutely hate the texture of hairless animals (makes me want to vomit), and I will 100% use gloves every time.

I am also very temperature sensitive, specifically to being overheated, and thus strip down to a tank top before scrubbing into surgery. Otherwise, I will get too hot and become decidedly unpleasant to be around.

Story B: Job Crafting as a Solution

Some parts of vet school were a struggle, specifically for sensory processing. Anatomy lab, group projects during class time. I never got much from them, and all of the chatter often triggered migraines. I also learned to wear earplugs on exam days to filter out background noise.

Now I'm a large animal vet. Being solo in the truck so much, and outside the rest of the time, is definitely my jam.

involved in empathy and self–other processing, whereas SPS is associated with heightened engagement of these same neural circuits (Acevedo et al. 2018). Differences also emerge in supportive contexts. In more positive environments, higher SPS is associated with greater well-being – a pattern that has not been observed for autism (Damatac et al. 2025).

This last finding once again highlights the duality of this personality trait. While some situations may prove more stressful for people with elevated SPS, in certain contexts, this trait can lead to higher well-being. To maximize the benefits of SPS, coping strategies and job crafting are essential. Creating roles or routines that reduce overstimulation, such as quiet spaces, scheduled breaks, or collaborative team structures, can protect well-being. Story 2.2 outlines different coping strategies used by a veterinarian in practice, as well as how another veterinarian found a good match to her sensory needs in her job as a large animal veterinarian, which is an example of job crafting. Some HSPs also benefit from boundary-setting, mindfulness practices, and tailoring work tasks to emphasize strengths such as empathy and attention to detail. While SPS can pose challenges, it can also foster deep compassion satisfaction and professional fulfillment when well-managed (Pérez-Chacón et al. 2021).

WORKAHOLISM

For many veterinary professionals, the work is not simply a job; it is a calling. A strong sense of purpose and commitment to animal care often drives individuals to enter and remain in the field, even in the face of stress and personal sacrifice. According to recent data, a majority of veterinary professionals report feeling a deep, vocational attachment to their work (Moody 2022). While this dedication can be a powerful motivator, it may also mask unhealthy work behaviors, particularly workaholism.

Workaholism refers to a compulsive need to work excessively and persistently, often at the expense of personal well-being. In veterinary medicine, the competitive nature of veterinary school admissions and the high demands of clinical training may attract or reinforce workaholic tendencies. The culture of veterinary education often normalizes overwork, fostering environments where long hours and emotional overextension are seen as signs of professional commitment (Steffey et al. 2023).

Story 2.3 provides a striking example of this progression. Early in their career, one clinician described how the long hours of veterinary training conditioned them to equate constant work with dedication. Even after completing residency, they continued to visit the clinic on days off,

STORY 2.3 WORKAHOLISM

Early in my career, I conditioned myself to work constantly. Starting during my clinical rotations in vet school, working seven days a week was just the norm. Days would often start at 6 am and frequently go late, sometimes until 9 pm. Veterinary medicine was my life. It was something I had strived for for so long that, at first, it almost seemed like a privilege to get to do the thing I loved so much every waking hour of the day. In retrospect, I sustained that work ethic far longer than I should have.

Even after I finished my residency and was in practice, I would still pop into the clinic on my days off to check on patients. I remember thinking that my new four-day-a-week schedule was a ridiculous luxury after years of grueling training. I literally didn't know what to do with my free time. I had no hobbies. I had nothing else, so naturally I just went to work. I would often be found in the clinic on my days off, checking on patients and calling owners. My dedication was noted and appreciated by my boss, reinforcing the behavior.

As the years went on, my dedication started to feel like a burden. I dreaded going to work at all, much less on my days off. I was bitter about coming in on my days off, even though literally no one had insisted I do so. About four years into practice, I finally hit a wall. My mental health was declining. I was burned out, depressed, and occasionally suicidal. I think those suicidal thoughts were actually what shook me out of it. Those thoughts made me realize just how miserable I was, prompting some big changes in my life. I quit my job and started working locum. The scarcity of my specialty meant I would fly to other states to work a week at a time, then come home for a week or so before returning. I purposefully limited my schedule and set strict boundaries for my time away from work. No emails, no phone calls on my days off. When I wasn't in the clinic, I wasn't in the clinic. I started to have hobbies again. I took classes and spent time with my spouse. I finally started to learn what balance meant. A few years later, a job opportunity presented itself close to home, and I was frankly sick of traveling. I am happy to say that I was able to maintain those boundaries as I settled into regular practice, and I am a much happier person for it.

unable to separate their identity from their professional role. Over time, what began as passion transformed into exhaustion and emotional collapse, culminating in burnout and suicidal ideation. The clinician ultimately regained well-being only after redefining boundaries, restricting work hours, taking time for recovery, and reclaiming a sense of life outside the clinic.

This story reflects patterns identified in the literature. Workaholism is understood as both a personality trait, linked to conscientiousness and perfectionism, and a cultural phenomenon reinforced by professional norms and expectations. While some level of work engagement can promote mastery and satisfaction, persistent overwork is associated with burnout, fatigue, emotional detachment, and reduced job satisfaction (Lakkawar et al. 2020). Over time, chronic overwork without adequate recovery can damage physical health, relationships, and career sustainability.

Addressing workaholism in veterinary medicine requires both individual and systemic strategies. Interventions include promoting work-life boundaries, encouraging time off, creating supportive workplace policies, and challenging the cultural glorification of overwork. Recognizing the difference between meaningful dedication and harmful overcommitment is essential to protecting the well-being of veterinary professionals (Sonnentag and Fritz 2015; Lakkawar et al. 2020; Steffey et al. 2023).

PLASTICITY, COPING, AND THE ROLE OF PERSONALITY IN WELL-BEING

In Chapter 1, we discussed briefly that happiness is partially determined by genetics. However, we did not discuss potential mechanisms for this observed pattern. Consideration of personality provides some of that context. Similar to Lykken's (1996) twin work on happiness, large-scale twin research into personality shows substantial heritability (often ~40%–60%) that can shift across the life span. Shared environmental effects typically decline with age, while non-shared environmental influences remain important (Kandler et al. 2021).

Neuroscientific findings are consistent with the patterns seen in twin research. Studies reveal shared genetic links between brain structure and personality traits (Valk et al. 2020), while environmental inputs – like stress or education – can influence brain development and, in turn, personality expression (Grazioplene and Allen 2021). This highlights how plasticity allows experiences to shape biologically rooted traits.

Critically, the boundary between genes and environment is often blurred. Environmental influences, such as the personality traits of the parents who raise you, may themselves be influenced by genetics (Hart et al. 2021), reinforcing the view that nature and nurture are interwoven. Modern approaches call for a shift beyond fixed personality traits toward understanding personality as a flexible, goal-directed system shaped by both biology and context (Bergner 2020; Dubois et al. 2020).

Although personality traits are often used to predict patterns in behavior and well-being, they are not fixed labels of "strength" or "weakness." Modern research emphasizes that personality is both relatively stable and changeable, shaped by life experiences, environments, and deliberate efforts (Bleidorn et al. 2020). Traits like conscientiousness, neuroticism, and extraversion interact dynamically with context and coping strategies, helping explain why no trait is inherently beneficial or harmful in isolation.

Let us return to neuroticism as an example. While often associated with emotional sensitivity and risk for anxiety or burnout, neuroticism can also foster vigilance, caution, and preparation, qualities that are vital in high-stakes settings like medicine. For example, in Story 2.4, a young veterinary clinician preparing to perform a complex, high-risk procedure let their anxiety fuel extensive research. When complications arose during the procedure, their preparedness saved the patient. While staying up late to study for cases isn't likely to be beneficial for long-term wellness, in this instance, neuroticism, often viewed as a liability, became a clinical asset.

Empirical research supports this dual view. Neuroticism is linked to negative affect (Giluk 2009) and increased psychological distress, but also predicts engagement with treatment and higher motivation to avoid errors (Bucher et al. 2019). Similarly, conscientiousness is associated with resilience and better health behaviors (Rhodes and Wilson 2020), but in excess, can contribute to rigidity or workaholism. These findings highlight that it is not the presence of a trait, but how it is managed, that determines its impact.

This is where coping and intervention come in. Personality traits may have biological and developmental roots, but they can be expressed in more or less adaptive ways. Various exercises have shown benefits in shaping how our personalities manifest in our daily lives. For example, mindfulness is a learned skill that buffers the emotional intensity associated with high neuroticism (Giluk 2009), while goal-setting and environmental design can reinforce the positive aspects of conscientiousness (Rhodes and Wilson 2020). Reflective practice, peer support, and skill-building interventions offer professionals tools to work with their traits rather than against them – amplifying their potential while reducing their risks. In veterinary medicine, this means well-being is not reserved for those with a "perfect" personality profile. Instead, it emerges from self-awareness, strategic coping, and a flexible approach to personal growth.

CONCLUSION

Throughout this chapter, we have discussed how personality traits influence our experiences and well-being. Traits such as neuroticism, conscientiousness, or empathy influence what we notice, how strongly we react, and how quickly we recover. Yet, these traits are not fixed labels, nor do they fully determine your destiny. Experiences, environment, and deliberate practice all shape their expression over time.

STORY 2.4 THE POSITIVE SIDE OF NEUROTICISM

Atlanto-axial luxation is a spinal condition in which the dens and ligaments of C2 are absent or otherwise compromised, which leads to poor attachment of C1 to C2. When patients bend their heads down, their spine luxates and crushes the spinal cord. The surgery to fix this is a dangerous and complicated procedure, with perioperative mortality rates reported as high as 20%. Patients are often tiny – sometimes less than a kilogram – and you have to place two screws precisely. The placement of the screws is mostly blind; you find your landmarks, and drill, praying that the dog doesn't jump because your drill just went through the spinal cord or hemorrhage because you hit the spinal artery. Combined with that, the patients are often young, and their bones aren't fully formed. Often, the consistency of vertebrae is more like firm cheddar than bone, and, like a nice firm cheddar, it can crack when pressure is applied.

So, suffice it to say, I was pretty nervous before performing my first procedure. Especially at that time in my life, my neurotic personality tended to drive rather obsessive and frenetic behavior. So the day before the procedure, late into the night, I obsessively read just about every paper and book chapter that had ever been written on the subject.

And boy am I glad I did. The next day in surgery, we try to place the first screw, and the soft bone cracks. Okay, no problem, this happens, and my mentor and I proceed to attempt the salvage procedure. Unfortunately, that breaks the bone again, as did the following technique we tried. After the third failure, my mentor looked at me with a bit of panic in his eyes. He didn't know what to do next, but I did. My neurotic reading the day before, my brain's tendency to not only envision the worst scenario, but also to plan for it, meant I knew another salvage procedure. The fourth procedure held, and we all held our breath as he woke up. But shortly thereafter, he started to breathe again on his own, which isn't guaranteed after you've broken C2 three different ways. We settled him into the ICU and said a little prayer.

I can't say I slept very well that night. I called in the ICU to check on the little guy a couple of times. The ICU techs were pretty used to that from me as I would often call in to check when my anxieties would keep me up at night. He did really well though, and went home walking for the first time in months at the end of the week. At discharge his owners even teased me about how worried I had been about their little guy. I remember them saying, "Look how great he looks! You were so worried, but you did such a good job!" I can't say that staying up until 2 am reading articles is the healthiest behavior, but in this case, it saved my patient's life. I've gotten much better at balancing my neurotic tendencies. Learning to accept both the good and the bad of that part of my personality was the first step in learning how to cope with them.

Individual impacts on well-being do not stop with personality traits. Other factors, such as a personal value structure – i.e. an individual's beliefs about what matters and what is right – also impact our perception of the world and, thereby, our well-being (Cake et al. 2015). Value congruence on topics, such as standards of animal welfare, client service ethos, boundaries, etc., between an individual and their work environment is also critical for well-being. A perceived misfit between value structures can amplify stress and reduce recovery time, especially among highly conscientious or empathic professionals (Crane et al. 2015). Individuals benefit from seeking roles that align with their values, and organizations benefit from designing roles and recruiting personnel that align with their values. This alignment can enhance meaning and retention (Cake et al. 2015; Crane et al. 2015).

Finally, there are a number of workplace stressors that influence our well-being. From things as straightforward as the hours we work to more complicated topics like moral distress, there are myriad stressors that veterinary professionals will have to navigate during their careers. Thankfully, there are also coping skills, supportive environments, and reflective practice that can strengthen resilience and help professionals thrive across their careers.

REFERENCES

Acevedo, B., Aron, E., Pospos, S., and Jessen, D. (2018). The functional highly sensitive brain: a review of the brain circuits underlying sensory processing sensitivity and seemingly related disorders. *Philosophical Transactions of the Royal Society B: Biological Sciences* 373 (1744): 20170161.

Aron, E.N. and Aron, A. (1997). Sensory-processing sensitivity and its relation to introversion and emotionality. *Journal of personality and social psychology* 73 (2): 345.

Aron, E.N., Aron, A., and Jagiellowicz, J. (2012). Sensory processing sensitivity: a review in the light of the evolution of biological responsivity. *Personality and Social Psychology Review* 16 (3): 262–282.

Atherton, G., Edisbury, E., Piovesan, A., and Cross, L. (2023). 'They ask no questions and pass no criticism': a mixed-methods study exploring pet ownership in autism. *Journal of Autism and Developmental Disorders* 53 (8): 3280–3294.

Bergner, R.M. (2020). What is personality? two myths and a definition. *New Ideas in Psychology* 57: 100759.

Bleidorn, W., Hopwood, C.J., Back, M.D. et al. (2020). Longitudinal experience-wide association studies—a framework for studying personality change. *European Journal of Personality* 34 (3): 285–300.

Boyle, G.J., Matthews, G., and Saklofske, D.H. (2008). Personality theories and models: An overview. In: *Personality Theory and Assessment: Personality Theories and Models*, vol. 1, 1. London, 29: SAGE.

Bucher, M.A., Suzuki, T., and Samuel, D.B. (2019). A meta-analytic review of personality traits and their associations with mental health treatment outcomes. *Clinical Psychology Review* 70: 51–63.

Cake, M.A., Bell, M.A., Bickley, N., and Bartram, D.J. (2015). The life of meaning: a model of the positive contributions to well-being from veterinary work. *Journal of Veterinary Medical Education* 42 (3): 184–193.

Cake, M.A., McArthur, M.M., Matthew, S.M., and Mansfield, C.F. (2017). Finding the balance: uncovering resilience in the veterinary literature. *Journal of Veterinary Medical Education* 44 (1): 95–105.

Capraro, R.M. and Capraro, M.M. (2002). Myers-Briggs Type Indicator score reliability across studies: a meta-analytic reliability generalization study. *Educational and Psychological Measurement* 62 (4): 590–602.

Cattell, H.E. and Mead, A.D. (2008). The sixteen personality factor. In: *The SAGE Handbook of Personality Theory and Assessment: Personality Measurement and Testing (Volume 2)*, vol. 2, 135. Los Angeles, London, New Delhi, Singapore: SAGE Publications Ltd.

Colombo, E.S., Crippa, F., Calderari, T., and Prato-Previde, E. (2017). Empathy toward animals and people: the role of gender and length of service in a sample of Italian veterinarians. *Journal of Veterinary Behavior* 17: 32–37.

Costa, P.T. and McCrae, R.R. (1992). *Revised NEO Personality Inventory (NEO-PI-R) and NEO Five-Factor Inventory (NEO-FFI): Professional Manual*. Odessa, FL: Psychological Assessment Resources.

Crane, M.F., Phillips, J.K., and Karin, E. (2015). Trait perfectionism strengthens the negative effects of moral stressors occurring in veterinary practice. *Australian Veterinary Journal* 93 (10): 354–360.

Damatac, Christienne G., Marleen J. ter Avest, Tom F. Wilderjans, et al. "Exploring sensory processing sensitivity: relationships with mental and somatic health, interactions with positive and negative environments, and evidence for differential susceptibility." *Current Research in Behavioral Sciences* 8 (2025): 100165.

Dawson, B.F. and Thompson, N.J. (2017). The effect of personality on occupational stress in veterinary surgeons. *Journal of Veterinary Medical Education* 44 (1): 72–83.

Derksen, F., Bensing, J., and Lagro-Janssen, A. (2013). Effectiveness of empathy in general practice: a systematic review. *British Journal of General Practice* 63 (606): e76–e84.

Dubois, J., Eberhardt, F., Paul, L.K., and Adolphs, R. (2020). Personality beyond taxonomy. *Nature Human. Behaviour* 4 (11): 1110–1117.

Eley, D.S., Cloninger, C.R., Walters, L., et al., 2013. The relationship between resilience and personality traits in doctors: implications for enhancing well-being. *PeerJ*, 1, p.e216.

Eysenck, H.J. (1967). *The Biological Basis of Personality*. Springfield, IL: Charles C Thomas.

Ghanim, D.A., Gadelrab, H.F., and Alnassar, H.A. (2025). The differential mediating effect of self-efficacy in the relationship between adaptive and maladaptive perfectionism and burnout among physicians in Kuwait. *Journal of the Social Sciences* 53 (3): 298–328.

Giluk, T.L. (2009). Mindfulness, Big Five personality, and affect: a meta-analysis. *Personality and Individual Differences* 47 (8): 805–811.

Goldberg, L.R. (1990). An alternative "description of personality": the Big-Five factor structure. *Journal of Personality and Social Psychology* 59 (6): 1216–1229.

Goswami, A. and Baksi, R. (2025). Perfectionism as a catalyst to anxiety and burnout: a study among students. *IJPS* 7 (1): 273–287.

Grazioplene, R.G. and Allen, T.A. (2021). The neurobiology of personality. *Current Opinion in Behavioral Sciences* 39: 26–32.

Guilera, T., Batalla, I., Forné, C., and Soler-González, J. (2019). Empathy and big five personality model in medical students and its relationship to gender and specialty preference: a cross-sectional study. *BMC medical education* 19 (1): 57.

Hart, S.A., Little, C., and van Bergen, E. (2021). Nurture might be nature: cautionary tales and proposed solutions. *NPJ Science of Learning* 6 (1): 2.

Holden, C.L. (2020). Characteristics of veterinary students: perfectionism, personality factors, and resilience. *Journal of Veterinary Medical Education* 47 (4): 488–496.

Hook, J.N., Hall, T.W., Davis, D.E. et al. (2021). The Enneagram: a systematic review of the literature and directions for future research. *Journal of Clinical Psychology* 77 (4): 865–883.

Kandler, C., Bratko, D., Butković, A., et al., 2021. How genetic and environmental variance in personality traits shift across the life span: Evidence from a cross-national twin study. *Journal of Personality and Social Psychology*, 121(5), p.1079.

Kanji, N., Coe, J.B., Adams, C.L., and Shaw, J.R. (2012). Effect of veterinarian-client-patient interactions on client adherence to dentistry and surgery recommendations in companion-animal practice. *Journal of the American Veterinary Medical Association* 240 (4): 427–436.

Karaffa, K.M., Hancock, T.S., and Sanford-Martens, T.C. (2024). Perfectionistic cognitions, self-compassion, and psychological distress among veterinary students. *Journal of College Student Mental Health* 1–24.

Karaffa, K.M., Meyer, A.T., and Sanford-Martens, T.C. (2025). Client characteristics and the effectiveness of embedded counseling services in a college of veterinary medicine. *Journal of Veterinary Medical Education* 52 (5): 682–696.

Kogan, L.R., Rishniw, M., Hellyer, P.W., and Schoenfeld-Tacher, R.M. (2018). Veterinarians' experiences with near misses and adverse events. *Journal of the American Veterinary Medical Association* 252 (5): 586–595.

Kuper, N., Modersitzki, N., Phan, L.V. and Rauthmann, J.F., 2021. The dynamics, processes, mechanisms, and functioning of personality: an overview of the field. *British Journal of Psychology*, 112(1), pp.1–51.

Lakkawar, A., Kumar, R., Uma, S. et al. (2020). Occupational stress and its management among veterinary professionals. *International Journal of Veterinary Science and Animal Husbandry* 5 (2): 29–32.

Leger, K.A., Charles, S.T., Turiano, N.A., and Almeida, D.M. (2016). Personality and stressor-related affect. *Journal of personality and social psychology* 111 (6): 917.

Lewis, E.G. and Cardwell, J.M. (2020). The Big Five personality traits, perfectionism and their association with mental health among UK students on professional degree programmes. *BMC Psychology* 8 (1): 1–10.

Li, R. (2023). Revisiting person–situation interactionism. *Nature Reviews Psychology* 2 (1): Article 6.

Listou Grimen, H. and Diseth, Å. (2016). Sensory processing sensitivity: factors of the highly sensitive person scale and their relationships to personality and subjective health complaints. *Perceptual and Motor Skills* 123 (3): 637–653.

Lykken, D. and Tellegen, A. (1996). Happiness is a stochastic phenomenon. *Psychological Science* 7 (3): 186–189.

McArthur, M.L., Learey, T.J., Jarden, A. et al. (2021). Resilience of veterinarians at different career stages: the role of self-efficacy, coping strategies and personal resources for resilience in veterinary practice. *Veterinary Record* 189 (12): e771.

Melchers, M.C., Li, M., Haas, B.W. et al. (2016). Similar personality patterns are associated with empathy in four different countries. *Frontiers in psychology* 7: 290.

Menor-Campos, D.J., Knight, S., Sánchez-Muñoz, C., and López-Rodríguez, R. (2019). Human-directed empathy and attitudes toward animal use: a survey of Spanish veterinary students. *Anthrozoös* 32 (4): 471–487.

Mezquita, L., Bravo, A. J., Morizot, J., Pilatti, A., Pearson, M. R., Ibáñez, M. I., . . . & Cross-Cultural Addictions Study Team (2019). Cross-cultural examination of the Big Five Personality Trait Short Questionnaire: Measurement invariance testing and associations with mental health. *PloS one* 14 (12): e0226223.

Moody, A.B. (2022). *The dark side of calling: a partial test of the work as calling theory (WCT) using the veterinarian occupational well-being study (VOWS).* Ph.D. thesis. Colorado State University.

Morellini, L., Izzo, A., Celeghin, A. et al. (2023). Sensory processing sensitivity and social pain: a hypothesis and theory. *Frontiers in Human Neuroscience* 17: 1135440.

Osborn, S.A., Brummel, B.J., and Walton, H.R. (2024). Trainer perspectives on personality-based group training: learning objectives, training outcomes, and best practice recommendations. *Consulting Psychology Journal* 76 (2): 197.

Pérez-Chacón, M., Chacón, A., Borda-Mas, M., and Avargues-Navarro, M.L. (2021). Sensory processing sensitivity and compassion satisfaction as risk/protective factors from burnout and compassion fatigue in healthcare and education professionals. *International Journal of Environmental Research and Public Health* 18 (2): 611.

Perret, J.L., Best, C.O., Coe, J.B. et al. (2020). Association of demographic, career, and lifestyle factors with resilience and association of resilience with mental health outcomes in veterinarians in Canada. *Journal of the American Veterinary Medical Association* 257 (10): 1057–1068.

Pittenger, D.J. (1993). The utility of the Myers-Briggs Type Indicator. *Review of Educational Research* 63 (4): 467–488.

Pizzolon, C.N., Coe, J.B., and Shaw, J.R. (2019). Evaluation of team effectiveness and personal empathy for associations with professional quality of life and job satisfaction in companion animal practice personnel. *Journal of the American Veterinary Medical Association* 254 (10): 1204–1217.

Platt, B., Hawton, K., Simkin, S., Dean, R. and Mellanby, R.J., 2012. Suicidality in the veterinary profession. *Crisis: The Journal of Crisis Intervention and Suicide Prevention. Advance article*, 1–10. https://doi.org/10.1027/0227-5910/a000143

Pluess, M., Assary, E., Lionetti, F. et al. (2018). Environmental sensitivity in children: development of the Highly Sensitive Child Scale and identification of sensitivity groups. *Developmental Psychology* 54 (1): 51.

Radisavljević, D., Rzepka, R., and Araki, K. (2023). Personality types and traits—examining and leveraging the relationship between different personality models for mutual prediction. *Applied Sciences* 13 (7): 4506.

Rhodes, R.E. and Wilson, K.E. (2020). Personality and physical activity. In: *The Routledge International Encyclopedia of Sport and Exercise Psychology* (ed. D. Hackfort and R.J. Schinke), 413–425. London: Routledge.

Rinjani, A. (2023). Comparing the Myers-Briggs Type Indicator (MBTI) and DISC personality tests: strengths, weaknesses, and applications. *Journal of Psychological Research and Practice* 5 (2): 45–58.

Rolland, J.P. (2002). The cross-cultural generalizability of the five-factor model of personality. In: *The Five-Factor Model of Personality Across Cultures* (ed. R.R. McCrae and J. Allik). Dordrecht: Kluwer Academic.

Rossier, J., Aluja, A., García, L.F. et al. (2007). The cross-cultural generalizability of Zuckerman's alternative five-factor model of personality. *Journal of Personality Assessment* 89 (2): 188–196.

Setti, A., Lionetti, F., Kagari, R. et al. (2022). The temperament trait of environmental sensitivity is associated with connectedness to nature and affinity to animals. *Heliyon* 8 (7): e09861.

Smith, M.M., Sherry, S.B., Vidovic, V. et al. (2019). Perfectionism and the five-factor model of personality: A meta-analytic review. *Personality and Social Psychology Review* 23 (4): 367–390.

Sonnentag, S. and Fritz, C. (2015). Recovery from job stress: the stressor-detachment model as an integrative framework. *Journal of Organizational Behavior* 36 (S1): S72–S103.

Ståhlberg, J., 2015. The relationships between perfectionism, achievement goal orientations, and goal setting. https://helda.helsinki.fi/server/api/core/bitstreams/02cc756c-63c3-423a-991b-13a95f9aea81/content

Steffey, M.A., Griffon, D.J., Risselada, M. et al. (2023). Veterinarian burnout demographics and organizational impacts: a narrative review. *Frontiers in Veterinary Science* 10: 1234567.

Stoeber, J. and Childs, J.H. (2011). Perfectionism. *Current Psychology* 30 (3): 159–172.

Strickhouser, J.E., Zell, E., and Krizan, Z. (2017). Does personality predict health and well-being? A meta-synthesis. *Health Psychology* 36 (8): 797–810.

Unjai, S., Forster, E.M., Mitchell, A.E., and Creedy, D.K. (2024). Interventions to promote resilience and passion for work in health settings: a mixed-methods systematic review. *International Journal of Nursing Studies Advances* 7: 100242.

Valk, S.L., Hoffstaedter, F., Camilleri, J.A. et al. (2020). Personality and local brain structure: their shared genetic basis and reproducibility. *NeuroImage* 220: 117067.

Varela, M. and Correia, I. (2023). Empathy and burnout in veterinarians and veterinary nurses: Identifying burnout protectors. *Anthrozoös* 36 (1): 15–34.

Volk, J.O., Schimmack, U., Strand, E.B., and Lord, L.K. (2019). Executive summary of the Merck Animal Health Veterinary Wellbeing Study. *Journal of the American Veterinary Medical Association* 254 (1): 66–73.

Volk, J.O., Schimmack, U., Strand, E.B., and Lord, L.K. (2021). Executive summary of the Merck Animal Health Veterinary Wellbeing Study III. *Journal of the American Veterinary Medical Association* 259 (3): 239–251.

Volk, J.O., Schimmack, U., Strand, E.B., and Lord, L.K. (2023). Executive summary of the Merck Animal Health Veterinary Wellbeing Study IV. *Journal of the American Veterinary Medical Association* 261 (13): 1457–1470.

Wilkinson, H., Whittington, R., Perry, L., and Eames, C. (2017). Examining the relationship between burnout and empathy in healthcare professionals: a systematic review. *Burnout Research* 6: 18–29.

Winter, R., Issa, E., Roberts, N. et al. (2020). Assessing the effect of empathy-enhancing interventions in health education and training: a systematic review of randomised controlled trials. *BMJ Open* 10 (9): e036470.

Diversity and Well-Being

CHAPTER 3

Elisabeth Cavallaro, MPH, MCHES, Sraavya Polisetti, and Lisa M. Greenhill, MPA, EdD

American Association of Veterinary Medical Colleges, Washington, DC, USA

INTRODUCTION

The last two chapters have explored the complex interplay of factors that influence well-being, ranging from genetic predispositions to the coping mechanisms individuals develop over time (Lyubomirsky 2007; Warr and Nielsen 2018). Demographic variables such as race, socioeconomic status, gender, sexuality, age, religion, and physical or mental health also have a substantial influence on overall well-being (Brown and Moloney 2019). Individuals belonging to historically minoritized and marginalized populations often face cumulative social, economic, and educational barriers that negatively affect well-being (Fagrell et al. 2019).

The term *minoritized* refers to groups that have been socially, politically, or economically devalued through systemic structures of power, regardless of their numerical representation within a population. *Marginalized* populations are those excluded from full participation in social, economic, or political life (Brown and Moloney 2019). These concepts are closely linked to the framework of intersectionality, which describes how the different parts of our identities (gender, sexuality, race, etc.) are interconnected and collectively shape lived experience (Crenshaw 1989).

This chapter examines how these intersecting identities and experiences influence the well-being of individuals within the veterinary profession.

DEMOGRAPHICS

Veterinary medicine has historically been one of the more homogenous health professions. Within the veterinary workforce, women comprise 65.7% of practicing veterinarians, and those identifying as White make up 87% of the profession (DataUSA n.d.). Similar trends are observed among support staff. According to the National Association of Veterinary Technicians in America, 94% of members identify as female and 89% as White (NAVTA 2024).

Although the profession remains demographically narrow, gradual shifts in racial/ethnic diversity are emerging. According to the 2024–2025 American Association of Veterinary Medical Colleges (AAVMC) survey, over a quarter of students self-identify as underrepresented racial/ethnic minorities (AAVMC 2025). These changes hold promise for broader representation in the years ahead. With this growing diversity comes an essential responsibility to examine how the multiple dimensions of personal identity shape individual experiences of well-being and influence veterinary professionals' engagement with well-being support. Historically, the health and well-being of underrepresented individuals have received limited attention within professional cultures (Fagrell et al. 2019). However, research indicates that the more marginalized identities an individual holds, the higher their likelihood of experiencing chronic health conditions, which in turn can diminish overall well-being (Robards et al. 2020).

The impact of intersectionality on well-being is also evident in work environments. As we will discuss in the upcoming chapters, numerous factors impact well-being outcomes for veterinary professionals. Marginalization and minoritization can contribute to and compound these risk factors. However, attention to overall fairness and inclusion in the workplace is positively associated with well-being, regardless of one's identities (Enchautegui-de-Jesús 2006). Further, individuals who move in diverse social circles and engage in diverse activities tend to have higher levels of well-being (Celikdemir and Katrinli 2020). Thus, professional environments that prioritize diversity and equitable, inclusive practices should achieve better overall outcomes for all work team members.

GENDER

According to AAVMC, over 80% of veterinary students identify as female (AAVMC 2025). Given that women now constitute the majority of veterinary professionals, it might be assumed that gender-based disparities in well-being would be minimal. However, this assumption discounts the persistent underrepresentation of women in leadership roles across the profession. A 2022 survey found that men were twice as likely to be practice owners as women, and women were similarly underrepresented in other leadership roles, including Chief Veterinary Officers, academic leadership positions, and veterinary journal editorships (Jelinski 2022; Stärk et al. 2022; Vezeau et al. 2024).

Gender bias continues to shape professional experiences in veterinary medicine. The British Veterinary Association's survey found that female veterinarians were less likely to be recognized for their clinical expertise, were paid less than men in comparable roles, and were offered fewer opportunities for advancement (Begeny and Ryan 2018). Story 3.1 further illustrates this dynamic, describing the experiences of a female specialist whose male resident had to confirm her expertise in order to build client trust. Such experiences are emblematic of broader inequities linked to lower negotiation confidence and reduced job satisfaction – factors that directly affect well-being. Even in professions where women are numerically dominant, subtle microaggressions and systemic disparities in pay and recognition persist (Archuleta et al. 2024). Quantitative analyses from the United States further support these findings, revealing that female veterinary practice owners earn significantly less than their male counterparts, even after controlling for experience, ownership status (solo vs partner), and specialty certification (Neill et al. 2021). Such inequities not only undermine professional satisfaction but also contribute to longer-term challenges in retention and well-being (Neill et al. 2021).

STORY 3.1 THE IMPACT OF COLLEAGUE ADVOCACY

I was about a year out of my residency and was now in charge of training residents at my new job. I was basically the same age as the residents I was teaching, and a few were older than me. Add to that, I was also quite young-looking for my age. Daily, I fielded incredulous questions about whether I was, in fact, old enough to be a doctor. I tried to shrug them off with little quips like "Thanks, I moisturize!" but it was draining to be constantly doubted.

One afternoon, I was explaining a complicated plan for a trauma case to a client. It was scary, life-or-death, expensive, and you could tell they were terrified. They kept looking to my resident, who is male and looked older, for reassurance. They were quite clearly checking with him to see if I was saying the correct things. Was it because I look young? Was it because I am female? Maybe both? It was pretty uncomfortable, but I was just trying to soldier through it and focus on the pet. Eventually, and I will forever be grateful to him for this, my resident said, "Hey, don't let my looks fool you, I'm here to learn from her. You should listen to what she's saying." It reset the tone of that room in a heartbeat. Now the clients trusted me and were paying attention. All it took was for him to call it out and support me. I would have never dreamed of asking him to do that, but he was and is a very stand-up guy.

Gendered well-being disparities are amplified among women who hold intersecting marginalized identities. In both human and veterinary health care, women of color report disproportionately high rates of discrimination, microaggressions, and threats to psychological safety (Myers et al. 2023; Summers et al. 2023; Wheeler et al. 2019). In a 2020 review, 62% of Black female human healthcare providers reported patient-based discrimination, compared with 31% of Asian, 20% of Hispanic, and 6% of White women (Filut et al. 2020). Such experiences erode professional authority and contribute to chronic stress and reduced well-being (Ahmad et al. 2022). Additionally, women with disabilities tend to earn less, have fewer opportunities for autonomous or creative work, and experience greater workplace stress than nondisabled women and men with disabilities, and these factors are all linked to higher levels of depressive symptoms (Brown and Moloney 2019). Recognizing that race, gender identity, sexuality, and disability intersect to produce distinct health outcomes, research and policy must move beyond treating women as a homogenous category (Etherington 2015).

Research suggests that those who identify as women generally tend to have higher frequencies of internalizing conditions such as depression and general psychological distress, when compared to men (Matud et al. 2019). This trend is reflected in the veterinary literature, with female veterinarians experiencing both higher rates of depression (36.7% vs 24.5%) and serious psychological distress (37.6% vs 29.7%) than their male counterparts (Nett et al. 2015; Pohl et al. 2022). That said, some research suggests that the actual rates of internalized mental health conditions, such as depression, in men may be underestimated, partly because of how these conditions are measured and because men often face stigma or barriers when seeking help (Smith et al. 2018). In contrast, men generally are more likely to exhibit externalizing responses to distress, such as aggression or substance misuse (Rosenfield and Mouzon 2012). It should be noted that in the veterinary profession, alcohol abuse is equally common or slightly more common in women (Harling et al. 2009; Neubauer et al. 2024). Additionally, not all aspects of masculinity have positive mental health impacts, as conformity to traditional masculine norms, including emotional restriction, self-reliance, and maintaining power over women, has been associated with poorer mental health outcomes in men (Wong et al. 2017).

SEXUAL AND GENDER DIVERSITY

In the United States, approximately 7.1% of people identify as lesbian, gay, bisexual, transgender, or another sexual or gender minority (Jones 2022). Comparable proportions are seen within veterinary education, where 6.5% of students identify as Lesbian Gay Bisexual Transgender Queer/Questioning (LGBTQ) + (Greenhill and Carmichael 2014). Similar to patterns in the broader population, LGBTQ+ individuals in veterinary medicine experience higher rates of mental health challenges and suicidal ideation, reflecting the cumulative impact of stigma and discrimination across social and institutional contexts (Haas et al. 2010; Valdiserri et al. 2019; CDC 2022; Chum et al., 2023). Lesbian, gay, and bisexual veterinarians report poorer mental well-being, and transgender and nonbinary colleagues experience the highest levels of depression and suicidal thoughts (Witte et al. 2020).

The culture of the learning and working environment strongly shapes these outcomes. Campus climate studies across US and UK veterinary programs reveal that LGBTQ+ students are less likely to have faculty or staff mentors, more likely to encounter homophobic language, and more frequently subjected to verbal harassment, most often from peers (Greenhill and Carmichael 2014; Witte et al. 2020). In professional practice, many veterinarians describe feeling somewhat more comfortable being open about their identities and encountering less overt hostility, though formal institutional supports and LGBTQ+-specific well-being resources remain limited (Timmenga et al. 2022).

Promoting inclusion requires more than tolerance – it depends on environments that affirm identity and belonging. Research across health professions indicates that inclusive policy frameworks, mentorship programs, and visible representation improve retention and well-being (Valdiserri et al. 2019; Timmenga et al. 2022). Affirming environments that encourage authenticity and connection to community also strengthen resilience and professional satisfaction (Vaughan and Rodriguez 2014).

RACE/ETHNICITY

Racial and ethnic diversity within veterinary medicine remains substantially lower than in other health professions. As of 2023, 76.5% of US veterinary students identify as White, compared with 43.9% of MD students (AAMC 2023; AAVMC 2023). Representation of Black, Hispanic, and Indigenous students has grown modestly but remains disproportionately low, with participation varying significantly across institutions (AAVMC 2023). Historical analyses suggest that structural barriers, including socioeconomic inequities, limited role models, and cultural disconnects, continue to restrict access to veterinary education and career advancement (Brocato 2017). These disparities persist within faculty and leadership positions, where racially minoritized professionals remain underrepresented and often experience additional barriers to mentorship, promotion, and belonging (Burkhard et al. 2022; Dusome 2024).

Research consistently demonstrates that racial and ethnic discrimination negatively affects well-being. Racially minoritized veterinarians report experiencing microaggressions, exclusion, and differential treatment, which contribute to reduced belonging and well-being (Summers et al. 2023; Nishi et al. 2024; Barnes et al. 2025). A 2021 survey by the British Veterinary Association found that 27% of veterinarians from racially minoritized backgrounds experienced discrimination at work, compared with 14% of White respondents, with over one-third identifying clients or pet owners as the primary source (BVA 2021). These findings mirror experiences in human health care, where discrimination and bias from patients are well-documented sources of stress and moral injury (Wittkower et al. 2021; Hamed et al. 2022).

The consequences of racism extend beyond workplace interactions. Intergenerational and collective trauma continue to shape health outcomes across communities of color (Kirkinis et al. 2018). For Black Americans, the enduring legacy of slavery and systemic racism influences both physical and psychological health, while pressure to assimilate into dominant cultural norms can exacerbate distress (Liu et al. 2019). Racial oppression also manifests physiologically. Communities facing chronic discrimination experience higher rates of poverty, trauma exposure, and post-traumatic stress disorder, all of which increase risks for substance use and related health conditions (Ravi et al. 2023). Among Indigenous peoples, centuries of cultural erasure, land dispossession, and state-sanctioned oppression have disrupted collective identity and contributed to disproportionately high rates of substance use disorder and suicide (Skewes and Blume 2019). Discriminatory beliefs within health care systems often compound these harms, as underlying racial trauma is rarely addressed in treatment (Richards 2021; Hamed et al. 2022).

The internalization of discrimination (i.e. believing unfair treatment is deserved) further erodes well-being, fostering low self-esteem, anxiety, and depression (Hughes et al. 2015). Yet, experiences of collective identity and community connection can buffer these harms. Social identity theory suggests that a strong sense of cultural belonging enhances resilience and provides meaning in the face of adversity (Tajfel and Turner 1986; Hughes et al. 2015). Within veterinary medicine, racially and ethnically diverse professionals often describe finding support and purpose through affinity groups, mentorship networks, and community engagement initiatives that center representation and mutual care (Chung and Armitage-Chan 2022; Summers et al. 2023). Pride VMC, an LGBTQIA affinity group, has a list of veterinary affinity groups on their website https://pridevmc.org/sibling-organizations/.

Efforts to address racial inequities within veterinary education and practice must therefore move beyond recruitment targets to encompass structural and psychological well-being. Inclusive policies, leadership accountability, and visible representation are essential for fostering equitable participation and promoting health across all identities (Burkhard et al. 2022; AAVMC 2022). By recognizing both the harms of systemic racism and the protective power of collective identity, the profession can move toward a more inclusive and resilient culture of well-being. We recognize that in the current sociopolitical climate, formal diversity, equity, and inclusion programming has become more difficult to implement and sustain in our universities, yet they are more important than ever before.

DISABILITY AND WELL-BEING

Disabilities may be visible or invisible, encompassing physical, sensory, cognitive, and psychological conditions that influence professional participation and well-being. Globally, an estimated 1.3 billion people, or about 16% of the world's population, live with a disability (World Health Organization 2023). Approximately 20% of US veterinary professionals responding to a national survey on demographics and mental health reported having a disability, while data from the AAVMC indicate that about 12% of veterinary students report a disability (Gleeson 2020; Scoresby et al. 2023). In the United Kingdom, 43.6% of respondents to a national survey (vet students, vet nursing students, veterinary surgeons, and veterinary nurses) reported a physical health condition, 38.5% a mental health condition, 60.6% a chronic health condition, and 29.8% as neurodivergent (Plowden et al. 2024). The exact definition of what constitutes varies from survey to survey, which explains the disparity in these statistics. Regardless, in a large-scale US survey of veterinary professionals, disability status was identified as a key predictor of psychological distress and suicidal thoughts, highlighting the elevated well-being risk associated with disability within the veterinary profession (Scoresby et al. 2023).

A central barrier to well-being for disabled professionals is *disablism*, or systemic discrimination against people with disabilities. The term *ableism*, defined as "discrimination in favor of able-bodied people" (OED 2024), is often criticized for centering nondisabled perspectives. In contrast, *disablism* more accurately describes the lived experience of discrimination (Gappmayer 2020). Exposure to disablism has been linked to lower well-being in adults (Emerson 2010). Recent data from the Royal College of Veterinary Surgeons (RCVS) and the British Veterinary Chronic Illness Support (BVCIS) initiative illustrate the scope of this issue in veterinary medicine. Over one-third of respondents (34.7%) reported being treated differently at work or during training because of their disability, most often due to visible symptoms or the act of disclosing their condition (Plowden et al. 2024). Among those who had disclosed, nearly half (45%) believed disclosure contributed to differential treatment, and only 45% felt their employer understood how their condition affected their work. Further findings from this survey are summarized in Table 3.1.

These findings reflect a broader pattern of disablism within health care professions, where structural and attitudinal barriers often undermine inclusion and well-being. The RCVS study further documented that 36% of veterinary professionals with disabilities experienced discrimination, bullying, or harassment, with higher rates among those with neurodivergent identities or mental health conditions. Comparable patterns are seen in broader US workforce data, where approximately one in three disabled employees reports workplace discrimination despite existing legal protections (Parisi 2024). Story 3.2 discusses the experiences of a vet student with dwarfism, and how they found both discriminatory and supportive environments during their career path.

Table 3.1 Experiences of disabled veterinary professionals (RCVS 2021).

Finding	Statistic	Context/Note
Reported being treated differently at work or during studies due to disability/ chronic condition	**34.7%**	Respondents commonly cited visible symptoms or the act of disclosure as triggers.
Believed disclosure contributed to differential treatment	**45.3%**	Many reported hesitation to disclose for fear of repercussions.
Felt their employer understood their condition	**45.2%**	Understanding decreased with a number or complexity of conditions.
Experienced discrimination, bullying, or harassment at work	**18.6%**	Highest among those with neurodivergent or mental health conditions.

Source: Adapted from Plowden Roberts et al., (2024).

STORY 3.2 THE IMPORTANCE OF ADVOCACY, AND INCLUSION IN THE WORKPLACE

I have dwarfism. When I was a senior in vet school, I was on the orthopedic surgical rotation. In order to be at the same level as the surgeon, I had to stand on a rickety stool on top of another bigger stool. I couldn't really shift my feet because I would potentially fall off. It was fine. I knew I needed to adapt to the surgeon.

However, that day the surgeon was a resident who was notoriously slow. It took them three hours to complete a TPLO. I was holding the stifle for hours while standing on the stools. He was getting frustrated and started blaming me for "moving too much." I couldn't feel my hands at that point, but I knew I was holding still. He kept getting angrier and angrier and finally told me to scrub out. He also said, "If you can't physically do stuff like this, you probably don't belong in this profession."

I was devastated. I already had so much doubt about my abilities, and this was my first rotation in my senior year. Thankfully, the surgery techs (who I worked with for a few summers) heard and saw what happened and marched right up to the Chief of Staff's office. He emailed me to talk about the incident. I thought I was going to be kicked out of school. Instead, he apologized profusely and told me I wasn't the problem.

Contrast that to my current boss, who spent thousands of dollars to get a hydraulic lift dental table for me. I seriously cried when I was able to do a procedure with my feet on the floor and not on a stool.

Disablism manifests in multiple ways, including inaccessible workplaces, infantilization, and implicit expectations that disabled professionals must adapt without structural support. Persistent exposure to these experiences contributes to poorer well-being outcomes and amplifies health inequities, particularly when intersecting with other marginalized identities such as race, gender, or sexuality (Branco et al. 2019).

Language and institutional culture can perpetuate exclusion. Disablist speech and the refusal of reasonable accommodations reinforce stigma and social withdrawal (Jóhannsdóttir et al. 2022). Accessibility gaps also extend into financial systems and well-being initiatives, where programs often presume able-bodied participation and frame accommodations as special requests rather than standard equity measures (Puli et al. 2024).

The effects of disablism may extend beyond individuals to families and caregivers, who experience secondary exposure to stigma and exclusion (Jarrett et al. 2014). For veterinary professionals, addressing these barriers requires not only policy change but also active engagement with universal design principles, accessibility audits, and leadership accountability to ensure that disability inclusion is embedded within the professional culture.

PROTECTIONS AND SYSTEMIC APPROACHES

Across identity groups, research consistently demonstrates that belonging and inclusion act as protective factors against psychological distress (Ellemers and Haslam 2012; Smith and Silva 2011). Social identity theory posits that identification with a group and positive in-group evaluation enhance self-esteem and buffer the adverse effects of discrimination (Tajfel et al. 2001). Within veterinary medicine, inclusive work environments, mentorship, and peer support networks can perform a similar function in mitigating the well-being impacts of marginalization (Enchautegui-de-Jesús et al. 2006; Timmenga et al. 2022).

Examples from professional experience illustrate how these mechanisms operate in practice. Story 3.1 describes a clinician whose authority was repeatedly questioned due to age and gender until a colleague explicitly affirmed her role in front of a client. This act of allyship restored

STORY 3.3 INCLUSIVE COMMUNICATION THROUGH CLINIC POLICY

As part of our new client paperwork, we have clients sign a behavior agreement. It says, "We understand that having a sick pet is a stressful time, and we are here to help. We promise to treat you with empathy, kindness and respect, and ask that you do the same for our team. Abusive language, threats, as well as homophobic, transphobic, racist or sexist language will not be tolerated and are grounds for removal from our practice."

When we put this policy in place, I honestly was just thinking about protecting my team from abusive clients. I wanted it to be crystal clear that we don't tolerate that sort of behavior right from the start. However, it had another effect I had not even considered. At the end of a consult, a client actually thanked me for the policy. They said that it immediately made them feel more welcome and comfortable as a trans person. I was so happy that we could make things just a little more comfortable for that pet owner.

professional credibility and demonstrated how social validation within teams can strengthen psychological safety.

Story 3.2 recounts the experience of a veterinary student with dwarfism who was unfairly criticized during surgery. Technicians who witnessed the incident intervened, reported the discriminatory behavior to the supervisor, and ensured the student received institutional support. Later in her career, the same individual found an inclusive workplace that provided adjustable equipment to facilitate participation in clinical work. This example underscores both the importance of bystander action and the tangible impact of accessible design on inclusion in everyday practice.

At the organizational level, policies that explicitly define behavioral expectations can foster both safety and a sense of belonging. Story 3.3 describes a clinic that implemented a client behavior policy prohibiting discriminatory language, which unexpectedly led a transgender client to express gratitude for feeling welcomed. Such initiatives reinforce inclusion as a collective norm rather than an individual burden.

Empirical evidence parallels these experiences. Close in-group ties and cross-cultural friendships each moderate the psychological impact of discrimination (Benner and Wang 2017). Affirming models of disability that reject deficit-based framing are linked with greater self-acceptance and agency (Silvers 2009; Wasserman and Aas 2023). Together, these findings underscore the protective value of belonging and equitable institutional design.

PROFESSIONAL RESPONSIBILITIES AND STRUCTURAL REFORM

Sustaining these protections requires systemic rather than individual approaches. The 2023 AAVMC *Exemplar for Technical Standards* outlines that essential veterinary competencies may be met with or without accommodations, reframing disability as a dimension of diversity rather than limitation (AAVMC 2023).

Academic and clinical institutions can further advance equity by:

- Conducting comprehensive audits of accessibility, policy, and inclusivity across learning and practice environments.
- Establishing formal mentorship and affinity networks for individuals from underrepresented backgrounds.
- Implementing transparent reporting mechanisms for discrimination and bias.
- Incorporating structured allyship and bystander intervention training.

These measures shift responsibility for well-being from individuals to organizations and help normalize inclusion as a professional standard.

CONCLUSION

Diversity and well-being are interdependent outcomes within veterinary medicine. Equitable systems that support representation, access, and inclusion contribute directly to professional sustainability. Individual resilience, while valuable, cannot compensate for structural inequity. Embedding inclusion into institutional culture ensures that all members of the profession can participate fully and safely.

REFERENCES

Ahmad, S.R., Ahmad, T.R., Balasubramanian, V. et al. (2022). Are you really the doctor? physician experiences with gendered microaggressions from patients. *Journal of Women's Health* 31 (4): 521–532.

American Association of Veterinary Medical Colleges (2022, April) Annual Data Report 2021-2022 [Internet]. Washington, DC. pp. 1–67. https://www.aavmc.org/about-aavmc/public-data/

American Association of Veterinary Medical Colleges (2023, March). Annual Data Report 2022-2023 [Internet]. Washington, DC: pp. 1–67. https://www.aavmc.org/about-aavmc/public-data/

American Association of Veterinary Medical Colleges (AAVMC), 2025. 2025 AAVMC Annual Data Report. https://www.aavmc.org/wp-content/uploads/2025/05/2025-AAVMC-Annual-Data-Report-Final.pdf (accessed 12 July 2025).

Archuleta, S., Ibrahim, H., Pereira, T.L.B., and Shorey, S. (2024). Microaggression interactions among healthcare professionals, trainees and students in the clinical environment: a mixed-studies review. *Trauma, Violence, & Abuse* 25 (1): 15248380241265380.

Association of American Medical Colleges (AAMC) (2023). 'Table B-5.1: Total Enrollment by U.S. MD-Granting Medical School and Race/Ethnicity (Alone), 2023-2024', 2023 FACTS: Enrollment, Graduates, and MD-PhD Data. Available at: https://www.aamc.org/media/6131/download (Accessed: 14 May 2026).

Barnes, K.H., Johnson, S., Liu, C.C., and Aulakh, K.S. (2025). Prevalence of mistreatment in veterinary medical education: a survey of 3rd year veterinary students at a single university. *BMC Medical Education* 25 (1): 305.

Begeny, C., Ryan, M., and with the British Veterinary Association (2018). *Gender Discrimination in the Veterinary Profession: A Brief Report of the BVA Employers' Study 2018*. London: British Veterinary Association.

Benner, A.D. and Wang, Y. (2017). Racial/ethnic discrimination and adolescents' well-being: The role of cross-ethnic friendships and friends' experiences of discrimination. *Child Development* 88 (2): 493–504.

Branco, C., Ramos, M.R. and Hewstone, M. (2019), The Association of Group-Based Discrimination with Health and Well-Being: A Comparison of Ableism with Other "Isms". Journal of Social Issues, 75: 814--846. https://doi.org/10.1111/josi.12340

British Veterinary Association (BVA). 2021. BVA discrimination in the veterinary profession statistics 2021. https://www.bva.co.uk/media/4393/bva-discrimination-stats-2021.pdf (accessed 1 December 2025).

Brocato, B.R. (2017). Why so white? A pilot study of the sociocultural factors influencing minority students' choice of veterinary medicine. PhD dissertation. College Station, TX: Texas A&M University. Available at: Texas A&M University OAKTrust Repository (Accessed: 14 May 2026).

Brown, R.L. and Moloney, M.E. (2019). Intersectionality, work, and well-being: the effects of gender and disability. *Gender & Society* 33 (1): 94–122.

Burkhard, M.J., Dawkins, S., Knoblaugh, S.E. et al. (2022). Supporting diversity, equity, inclusion, and belonging to strengthen and position the veterinary profession for service, sustainability, excellence, and impact. *Journal of the American Veterinary Medical Association* 260 (11): pp. 1283–1290. doi: 10.2460/javma.21.11.0477.

Celikdemir, D.Z., Katrinli, A. (2020). Efficient diversity management for workplace well- being. In: Dhiman, S. (eds) The Palgrave Handbook of Workplace Well-Being. Palgrave Macmillan, Cham. https://doi.org/10.1007/978-3-030-02470-3_5-1

Centers for Disease Control and Prevention. 2022, July 19. Suicide and violence prevention among gay and bisexual men. https://www.cdc.gov/msmhealth/suicide-violence-prevention.htm (accessed 21 February 2024).

Chum A, Kim C, Nielsen A, et al. Disparities in suicide-related behaviors across sexual orientations by gender: a retrospective cohort study using linked Health Administrative Data. *American Journal of Psychiatry*. 2023;180(9):660–667. doi:https://doi.org/10.1176/appi.ajp.20220763

Chung, G.H. and Armitage-Chan, E. (2022). Student experience and ethnic diversity: the experiences of underrepresented minority students at a veterinary university in the United Kingdom. *Journal of Veterinary Medical Education* 49 (3): 363–371.

Crenshaw, K. (1989). Demarginalizing the Intersection of Race and Sex: A Black Feminist Critique of Antidiscrimination Doctrine. *University of Chicago Legal Forum* 1989: 139–168.

DataUSA, n.d. Veterinarians: race and ethnicity profile. https://datausa.io/profile/soc/veterinarians?races-filter=shareR (accessed 14 December 2025).

Dusome, K. (2024). *Investigating Representations and Students' Challenges, Experiences and Perceptions of Equity, Diversity and Inclusion at Veterinary Colleges in Canada and the USA* (Doctoral dissertation,. University of Guelph).

Ellemers, N. and Haslam, S.A. (2012). Social identity theory. In: *Handbook of Theories of Social Psychology* (ed. P.A.M. Van Lange, A.W. Kruglanski, and E.T. Higgins), 379–398. London, Thousand Oaks, New Delhi: Sage Publications Ltd. https://doi.org/10.4135/9781446249222.n45.

Emerson E. Self-reported exposure to disablism is associated with poorer self-reported health and well-being among adults with intellectual disabilities in England: a cross-sectional survey. Public Health 2010, December; 124(12):682–9. doi:https://doi.org/10.1016/j.puhe.2010.08.020.

Enchautegui-de-Jesús, N., Hughes, D., Johnston, K.E., and Oh, H.J. (2006). Well-being in the context of workplace ethnic diversity. *Journal of Community Psychology* 34 (2): 211–223.

Etherington, C. (2015). Race, gender, and the resources that matter: an investigation of intersectionality and health. *Women & Health* 55 (7): 754–777.

Fagrell Trygg, N., Gustafsson, P.E., and Månsdotter, A. (2019). Languishing in the crossroad? a scoping review of intersectional inequalities in mental health. *International Journal for Equity in Health* 18 (1): 1–13.

Filut, A., Alvarez, M., and Carnes, M. (2020). Discrimination toward physicians of color: a systematic review. *Journal of the National Medical Association* 112 (2): 117–140.

Gappmayer, G. (2020). Disentangling disablism and ableism: the social norm of being able and its influence on social interactions with people with intellectual disabilities. Journal of Occupational Science, 28(1), 102–113. https://doi.org/10.1080/14427591.2020.1814394

Gleeson, M. (2020). Veterinary schools rethink standards for students with physical disabilities. *INSIGHT Into Academia* May 18. https://insightintoacademia.com/veterinary-schools-rethink-standards-for-students-with-physical-disabilities/.

Greenhill LM, Carmichael KP. Survey of college climates at all 28 US colleges and Schools of Veterinary Medicine: preliminary findings. Journal of Veterinary Medical Education. 2014;41(2):111–121. doi:https://doi.org/10.3138/jvme.0513-075r1

Haas AP, Eliason M, Mays VM, et al. Suicide and suicide risk in lesbian, gay, bisexual, and transgender populations: review and recommendations. *Journal of Homosexuality*. 2010;58(1):10–51. doi:https://doi.org/10.1080/00918369.2011.534038

Hamed, S., Bradby, H., Ahlberg, B.M., and Tholin, A. (2022). Racism in healthcare: a scoping review. *BMC Public Health* 22: 1602.

Harling, M., Strehmel, P., Schablon, A., and Nienhaus, A. (2009). Psychosocial stress, demoralization and the consumption of tobacco, alcohol and medical drugs by veterinarians. *Journal of Occupational Medicine and Toxicology* 4 (1): 4.

Hughes, M., Kiecolt, K.J., Keith, V.M., and Demo, D.H. (2015). Racial identity and well-being among African Americans. *Social Psychology Quarterly* 78 (1): 25–48. https://doi.org/10.1177/0190272514554043.

Jarrett, C.F., Mayes, R., and Llewellyn, G. (2014). The impact of disablism on the psycho-emotional well-being of families with a child with impairment. *Scandinavian Journal of Disability Research* 16 (3): 195–210.

Jelinski, M.D., Schreiner, B., Neale, A., and Townsend, H.G. (2022). Demographic survey of private veterinary practices in western Canada. *The Canadian Veterinary Journal* 63 (1): 27.

Jóhannsdóttir, Á., Egilson, S. Þ., & Haraldsdóttir, F. Implications of internalised ableism for the health and wellbeing of disabled young people. Sociology of Health & Illness 2022; 44: 360–376. https://doi.org/10.1111/1467-9566.13425

Jones, J.M. (2022, February 17.). LGBT identification in U.S. ticks up to 7.1%. *Gallup.com* https://news.gallup.com/poll/389792/lgbt-identification-ticks-up.aspx.

Kirkinis, K., Pieterse, A. L., Martin, C., et al. (2018). Racism, racial discrimination, and trauma: a systematic review of the social science literature. Ethnicity & Health, 26(3), 392–412. https://doi.org/10.1080/13557858.2018.1514453

Liu, W. M., Liu, R. Z., Garrison, Y. L., et al. (2019). Racial trauma, microaggressions, and becoming racially innocuous: the role of acculturation and White supremacist ideology. American Psychologist, 74(1), 143–155. https://doi.org/10.1037/amp0000368

Lyubomirsky S (2007) The How of Happiness: A New Approach to Getting the Life You Want. Penguin Press, New York. pg 37

Matud, M.P., López-Curbelo, M., and Fortes, D. (2019). Gender and psychological well-being. *International Journal of Environmental Research and Public Health* 16 (19): 3531.

Merriam-Webster. (n.d.). Ableism. In Merriam-Webster.com Dictionary. Retrieved August 11, 2024, from https://www.merriam-webster.com/dictionary/ableism

Myers, A.K., Williams, M.S., and Pekmezaris, R. (2023). Intersectionality and its impact on microaggression in female physicians in academic medicine: a cross-sectional study. *Women's Health Reports* 4 (1): 298–304.

National Association of Veterinary Technicians in America (NAVTA) 2024, NAVTA demographic survey results 2024: title protection, income, role clarity, and wellness within the veterinary technician profession, NAVTA. https://navta.net/documents-and-reports/. Accessed on March 28, 2026

Neill, C.L., Kakpo, A.T., and Mack, R. (2021). The role of experience, specialty certification, and practice ownership in the gender wage gap for veterinarians in the United States. *Journal of the American Veterinary Medical Association* 258 (6): 591–600.

Nett, R.J., Witte, T.K., Holzbauer, S.M. et al. (2015). Risk factors for suicide, attitudes toward mental illness, and practice-related stressors among US veterinarians. *Journal of the American Veterinary Medical Association* 247 (8): 945–955.

Neubauer, V., Dale, R., Probst, T., et al., 2024. Prevalence of mental health symptoms in Austrian veterinarians and examination of influencing factors. *Scientific Reports*, 14(1), p.13274.

Nishi, N.W., Collier, M.J., Morales, G.I., and Watley, E. (2024). Microaggressions in veterinary communication: what are they? How are they harmful? What can veterinary professionals and educators do? *Journal of the American Veterinary Medical Association* 262 (3): 1–6.

Oxford English Dictionary. (n.d.). Oxford English Dictionary. Retrieved August 11, 2024, from https://www.oed.com/.

Parisi, K. (2024, March 5). Exclusive: 25% of disabled workers have experienced discrimination during the job interview process, New Survey finds. *HR Brew* https://www.hr-brew.com/stories/2024/03/05/exclusive-25-of-disabled-workers-have-experienced-discrimination-during-the-job-interview-process-new-survey-finds.

Plowden Roberts, C., Robinson, D., and Rosolin, B. (2024). *Disability and Chronic Illness in Veterinary Work and Education: Full Report.* Brighton: Institute for Employment Studies, conducted on behalf of the Royal College of Veterinary Surgeons and British Veterinary Chronic Illness Support. https://www.rcvs.org.uk/news-and-views/publications/disability-and-chronic-illness-survey-full-report-final/disability-and-chronic-illness-survey-full-report.pdf.

Pohl, S., Möstl, E., Watzinger, F., Deeg, C. & Wagner, K.H., 2022. Stress and strain among veterinarians: a scoping review. *Irish Veterinary Journal*, 75(1), p.17. https://doi.org/10.1186/s13620-022-00220-x.

Puli L, Layton N, Bell D, Shahriar AZ. Financial inclusion for people with disability: a scoping review. Global Health Action. 2024, December 31;17(1):2342634. doi:https://doi.org/10.1080/16549716.2024.2342634.

Ravi, M., Mekawi, Y., Blevins, E.J. et al. (2023). Intersections of oppression: examining the interactive effect of racial discrimination and neighborhood poverty on PTSD symptoms in Black women. *Journal of Psychopathology and Clinical Science* 132 (5): 567.

Richards, D. (Center for Health Care Strategies), 2021. Incorporating racial equity into trauma-informed care. https://www.chcs.org/media/Brief-Incorporating-Racial-Equity-into-Trauma-Informed-Care.pdf

Robards F, Kang M, Luscombe G, et al. Intersectionality: social marginalisation and self-reported health status in young people. International Journal of Environmental Research and Public Health. 2020; 17(21):8104. https://doi.org/10.3390/ijerph17218104

Rosenfield, S., Mouzon, D. (2012). Gender and mental health. In: Aneshensel, C.S., Phelan, J.C., Bierman, A. (eds) Handbook of the Sociology of Mental Health: Handbooks of Sociology and Social Research. Springer, Dordrecht. https://doi.org/10.1007/978-94-007-4276-5_14

Scoresby, K., Jurney, C., Fackler, A. et al. (2023). Relationships between diversity demographics, psychological distress, and suicidal thinking in the veterinary profession: a nationwide cross-sectional study during COVID-19. *Frontiers in Veterinary Science* 10: 1130826.

Silvers, A. (2009). An essay on modeling: the social model of disability. In: Ralston, D., Ho, J. (eds.) Philosophical Reflections on Disability: Philosophy and Medicine, vol 104. Springer, Dordrecht. https://doi.org/10.1007/978-90-481-2477-0_2

Skewes, M. C., & Blume, A. W. (2019). Understanding the link between racial trauma and substance use among American Indians. American Psychologist, 74(1), 88–100. https://doi.org/10.1037/amp0000331

Smith, T.B. and Silva, L. (2011 Jan). Ethnic identity and personal well-being of people of color: a meta- analysis. *Journal of Counseling Psychology* 58 (1): 42–60. https://doi.org/10.1037/a0021528. PMID: 21171745.

Smith, D.T., Mouzon, D.M., and Elliott, M. (2018). Reviewing the assumptions about men's mental health: An exploration of the gender binary. *American journal of men's health* 12 (1): 78–89.

Stärk, K. D. C., Sifford, R. & van Andel, M. (2022) 'Who wants to be a chief veterinary officer (CVO)? – Thoughts on promoting leadership diversity in the public veterinary sector', *Frontiers in Veterinary Science*, 9: 937718. doi:https://doi.org/10.3389/fvets.2022.937718

Summers, O.S., Medcalf, R., Hubbard, K.A., and McCarroll, C.S. (2023). A cross-sectional study examining perceptions of discriminatory behaviors experienced and witnessed by veterinary students undertaking clinical extra-mural studies. *Frontiers in Veterinary Science* 10: 940836.

Tajfel, H. and Turner, J.C. (1986). The social identity theory of intergroup behaviour. *Psychology of intergroup relations* 2: 7–24.

Tajfel, H., Turner, J., Austin, W.G. and Worchel, S., 2001. An integrative theory of intergroup conflict. *Intergroup Relations: Essential Readings*, pp.94–109. Psychology Press. Philadelphia, PA

Timmenga FS, Jansen W, Turner PV, De Briyne N. Mental well-being and diversity, equity, and inclusiveness in the veterinary profession: pathways to a more resilient profession. Frontiers in Veterinary Science 2022;9. doi:https://doi.org/10.3389/fvets.2022.888189

Valdiserri, R.O., Holtgrave, D.R., Poteat, T.C., and Beyrer, C. (2019). Unraveling health disparities among sexual and gender minorities: a commentary on the persistent impact of stigma. *Journal of Homosexuality* 66 (5): 571–589.

Vaughan MD, Rodriguez EM. LGBT strengths: Incorporating positive psychology into theory, research, training, and practice. *Psychology of Sexual Orientation and Gender Diversity* 2014;1(4):325–334. doi:https://doi.org/10.1037/sgd0000053

Vezeau, N., Kemelmakher, H., Silva Seixas, J. et al. (2024). Characterizing global gender representation in veterinary executive leadership. *Journal of Veterinary Medical Education* 52 (1): 132–138.

Warr, P. and Nielsen, K. (2018). *Wellbeing and Work Performance: Handbook of Well-being*. Salt Lake City, UT: DEF Publishers.

Wasserman, David and Sean Aas, "Disability: definitions and models", *The Stanford Encyclopedia of Philosophy* (Fall 2023 Edition), Edward N. Zalta & Uri Nodelman (eds.), https://plato.stanford.edu/archives/fall2023/entries/disability/

Wheeler, M., de Bourmont, S., Paul-Emile, K. et al. (2019). Physician and trainee experiences with patient bias. *JAMA internal medicine* 179 (12): 1678–1685.

Witte, T.K., Kramper, S., Carmichael, K.P., Chaddock, M. and Gorczyca, K. (2020). A survey of negative mental health outcomes, workplace and school climate, and identity disclosure for lesbian, gay, bisexual, transgender, queer, questioning, and asexual veterinary professionals and students in the United States and United Kingdom. *Journal of the American Veterinary Medical Association* 257 (4): pp.417–431.

Wittkower, D., Bryan, J., and Asghar-Ali, A. (2021). Policies, recommendations and training to respond to patient microaggressions and hate speech aimed at healthcare professionals: a systematic review. *European Psychiatry* 64 (S1): S384–S384.

Wong, Y. J., Ho, M.-H. R., Wang, S.-Y., & Miller, I. S. K. (2017). Meta-analyses of the relationship between conformity to masculine norms and mental health-related outcomes. *Journal of Counseling Psychology*, 64(1), 80–93. https://doi.org/10.1037/cou0000176

World Health Organization (2023, March 7). Disability. In: *World Health Organization Fact Sheets*. https://www.who.int/news-room/fact-sheets/detail/disability-and-health.

CHAPTER 4 Mental Health

Carrie Jurney, DVM, DACVIM (Neurology)[1], Katie Lawlor, Psy.D[1], and Zachary Ward, PhD[2]

[1] *Not One More Vet, Inc, San Francisco, CA, USA*

[2] *School of Veterinary Medicine, University of California Davis, Davis, CA, USA*

THE INTERSECTION OF MENTAL HEALTH AND WELL-BEING

Well-being and mental health are interconnected yet distinct concepts; despite decades of research and discussion, there is no universally accepted definition of either. According to Michaelson et al. (2012), well-being encompasses how individuals feel and function on personal and social levels, and how they evaluate their overall lives. Mental health, while sharing similarities with well-being in addressing the emotional and psychological state of an individual, also involves the diagnosis and treatment of mental disorders (Balch et al. 2022).

The Diagnostic and Statistical Manual of Mental Disorders, Fifth Edition (DSM-5), a text used by mental health professionals in the diagnosis and treatment of mental health conditions, defines a mental disorder as "a syndrome characterized by clinically significant disturbance in an individual's cognition, emotion regulation, or behavior that reflects a dysfunction in the psychological, biological, or developmental processes underlying mental functioning. Mental disorders are usually associated with significant distress or disability in social, occupational, or other important activities" (American Psychiatric Association 2022).

Authors such as Stein (2021) underline that it is a combination of psychobiological dysfunction, as well as harm (i.e. impairment in important activities of living), that defines a disorder. Stein, much like the DSM-5, also notes that mental disorders are dynamic entities, subject to continual reevaluation as societal perspectives evolve. The harm caused by some conditions is extrinsic, due to stigmatization and societal rejection, rather than intrinsic. As our culture evolves, these harmful consequences resolve independently of individual efforts. For instance, homosexuality was listed as a mental disorder in earlier versions of the DSM, but as cultural progress has come to see homosexuality as a normal variation of sexuality, it is no longer listed as such.

Furthermore, many conditions are increasingly viewed on a spectrum of normality. For example, neurodevelopmental disorders, such as autism and attention-deficit/hyperactivity disorder (ADHD), have both psychobiological origins and social impacts, and therefore meet the criteria of a mental disorder. Additionally, many individuals seek medical care for neurodevelopmental disorders; however, with cultural shifts, these conditions are increasingly viewed as a spectrum of normality under the term "neurodiversity" rather than a "disorder" (Stein et al. 2021). Further blurring the lines, although concerns such as occupational stress, compassion fatigue, and burnout impact emotional states significantly, they are not considered mental disorders as they are generated by extrinsic stressors. However, associations between these external stressors and mental health conditions such as depression and anxiety have been widely documented, including within the field of veterinary medicine (Pohl et al. 2022).

All of this is to say that, as with so many aspects of medicine, biological organisms do not strictly adhere to the classification systems we try to place on them. A person does not have a mental health disorder like depression in a vacuum, and variables such as burnout may very well be part of their psychological state. Treatment of this person could involve medication, therapy, and/or adjustments to lifestyle. These interventions are not mutually exclusive; in fact, they work best in concert with each other.

The labels applied to our concerns have some utility, as they can help us in recognition and treatment approaches. However, when looking at ourselves or others, we should use a holistic lens, rather than reduce psychological health to a list of conditions. To this point, there has been a notable and sizable shift in recent years to the nomenclature and framework used by mental health professionals from discussing mental illness to emphasizing mental health. Underlying this change is an acknowledgment of the importance of a more comprehensive, positive, and proactive approach to psychological well-being (Balch et al. 2022).

This chapter will discuss the prevalence and statistics around mental health in the veterinary medicine community, as well as provide baseline information about mental health. The intention of this text is not to encourage self-diagnosis, but rather to empower veterinary professionals to find effective, evidence-based mental health care that meets their needs.

Discussions of well-being skills and interventions can be found in Chapter 10.

MENTAL HEALTH IN VETERINARY MEDICINE

The very existence of this textbook underscores the struggles with mental health within the field of veterinary medicine, a fact corroborated by existing literature. For example, specific mental health conditions, most often anxiety and depression-related, have been evaluated in the population. Elevated rates of anxiety are reported in about a quarter to a third of veterinary populations (Bartram et al. 2009; Best et al. 2020). Current rates of depression, while generally elevated compared to the general population, range widely from 6% to 28%, with approximately one third reporting depression at some point in their careers (Bartram et al. 2009; Best et al. 2020; Nett et al. 2015). For example, in a 2020 study of 3,118 German veterinarians, 27.78% screened positive for depression, compared with 3.99% of the general population (Schwerdtfeger et al. 2020).

A majority of papers engaging veterinary professionals are found to have elevated rates of various psychological concerns. The Kessler-6 inventory of psychological distress, a widely used assessment measuring levels of psychological distress and mental illness, has been used in multiple studies of veterinary mental health and well-being (da Silva et al. 2023; Mykyta 2023). According to researchers' findings, veterinary professionals are shown to have elevated rates of serious psychological distress, which is defined as distress that includes mental health problems severe enough to cause moderate-to-serious impairment in social and occupational functioning, and will require mental health care to resolve (Mykyta 2023; Scoresby et al. 2023; Volk et al. 2022).

With regard to suicidality, concerns among veterinarians are evident as early as a study of California veterinarians' mortality from 1960 to 1992. Within this population, compared to the general population, male veterinarians were 2.5 times more likely to die by suicide, and female veterinarians were 5.9 times more likely (Miller and Beaumont 1995). While somewhat improved from the initial numbers, a more recent US-based study shows a continued elevation in risk, with male and female veterinarians being at 1.6 and 2.4 times the risk, respectively (Witte et al. 2019). On a global scale, elevated rates of suicidal thoughts and actions in veterinarians have been documented in Germany, United States, Norway, the United Kingdom, and Australia (da Silva et al. 2023).

In recent years, the mental health of veterinary support staff has become a focus. Unfortunately, many of these studies find that support staff face psychological concerns equal to or even higher than those of their veterinarian counterparts (Scoresby et al. 2023; Witte et al. 2019; Volk 2022). In 2021, a survey of veterinary professionals was performed to assess the relation between various demographic factors, including job role, and both psychological distress and suicidal behavior. While the entire population of veterinary professionals had higher levels of serious psychological distress than the general public (2.7%), customer service representatives, veterinary assistants, and technicians all had elevated levels (54.1%, 57.8%, 48.0%), compared to associate veterinarians and practice owners

(28.6, 28.9%; Scoresby et al. 2023). The reason for this disparity is multifactorial, and this analysis showed that a variety of demographic factors, including gender, social class, age, and disability status, were all predictors of psychological distress in veterinary professionals (Scoresby et al. 2023).

BARRIERS TO MENTAL HEALTH CARE

Part of a holistic approach to mental health is seeking care when it would be beneficial. In the previous section, we discussed the prevalence of serious psychological distress. By definition, this type of distress includes mental health problems that are consequential enough to require treatment for recovery (Mykyta 2023).

In a study of US veterinarians performed in 2014, only 41% of veterinarians in serious psychological distress sought mental health care (Net 2015). In a 2022 study of US veterinary professionals, 59% of veterinarians and 65% of support staff with distress identified that they needed mental health care, but did not get it (Volk et al. 2022). This data begs the question—what is keeping people who clearly need—and even want—mental health care from receiving it?

In this section, we will discuss some barriers to mental health care and how to overcome them.

STIGMA

Studies have shown that 70–89% of US veterinarians believe that mental health treatment helps people live normal lives (Nett 2105; Volk et al. 2022). While these levels are lower than reported amongst the general public (93%), they still represent a substantial majority of veterinarians who support mental health care (Nett 2015). On a personal level, a majority of veterinarians (58%) also feel comfortable discussing mental health care with colleagues (Volk et al. 2022). Thus, on the surface, it would appear that the profession is largely supportive toward those experiencing mental health concerns.

Unfortunately, this is not the whole story. Significant stigma in seeking care remains prevalent within several populations in veterinary medicine. For instance, male veterinarians with 10–19 years of practice, as well as solo practitioners, are likely to display negative attitudes toward treatment effectiveness (Kassem et al. 2019). Additionally, multiple studies have found that people with serious psychological distress and suicidal ideation exhibit more negative perceptions of care and believe others will treat them more negatively for seeking help (Kassem et al. 2019; Nett et al. 2015; Volk et al. 2022). Indeed, only a minority of veterinarians in serious psychological distress agreed that they would feel comfortable taking time off to engage in treatment (22%) or that their practice management would be supportive of that type of care (25%), compared to 55% and 66% of nondistressed people (Volk et al. 2022). A significantly higher percentage of veterinarians (47.3%) were concerned about social judgments of receiving care than the much smaller percentage who were skeptical about treatment effectiveness (3.1%). This is unfortunate because, as discussed above, the vast majority of veterinarians support mental health care (Kassem et al. 2019; Volk et al. 2022). These barriers to engagement can potentially lead to a dire scenario, in which the people who need mental health care the most do not seek it out.

Combating mental health stigma necessitates a multifaceted approach. This involves education to dispel myths and fostering supportive environments that encourage a culture of acceptance and compassion. By embracing these strategies, we can break down barriers to care while ensuring that everyone has access to the support they need to thrive.

LICENSURE CONCERNS

Another barrier to treatment for healthcare professionals is concern over licensure and professional repercussions. This concern extends to both mental health conditions in general and specifically substance abuse. Although mental health concerns such as anxiety and depression are well-documented in the profession, substance-use behaviors are less frequently studied. In one German cohort of veterinary professionals, 57.4% reported using a psychoactive substance at some point in their careers, only 5% of which was prescribed by a medical professional (Harling et al. 2009). Access and diversion are risk factors for abuse, and a survey of Colorado veterinarians found that 12% were aware of veterinary staff opioid use and diversion (Mason et al. 2018). Alcohol is the most commonly abused substance, with various reports showing that about a quarter of veterinarians engage in binge drinking at least once a month (Harling et al. 2009; Volk et al. 2022). Although quantitative data is limited in the veterinary field, research has found fear of repercussions to one's job or license was a major factor associated with avoiding care for substance use and mental health conditions in human healthcare professionals, with up to 40% reporting reluctance to seek care due to these concerns (Dyrbye et al. 2017).

These fears are not unfounded. Historically, many veterinary licensing applications included questions about past mental illness or substance use, rather than focusing on current impairment, which is the recommended best practice. While most states have now transitioned to impairment-based questions, the lingering perception of risk continues to discourage some veterinarians from pursuing needed care (Cormier and Seddon 2024).

To address these barriers, the American Association of State Veterinary Boards (AASVB) recommends the creation of safe haven programs, which would allow veterinary professionals to self-report concerns confidentially and receive nondisciplinary treatment and monitoring. Some states have adopted these programs, but it is not yet a widespread practice. Evidence from similar programs in other healthcare professions shows these approaches are highly effective. A meta-analysis of over 3,000 human healthcare providers in substance abuse treatment found that 72% remained abstinent and 77% retained employment after participation in a monitoring program. These outcomes are approximately 1.5 times better than those in general substance-use treatment populations (Geuijen et al. 2021). These findings underscore that when clinicians are offered supportive, confidential pathways to recovery, rather than punitive oversight, they are far more likely to engage in care and achieve lasting success.

SOCIOCULTURAL BARRIERS

Culture reflects the shared beliefs and practices of a group of people. These ideas are often so ingrained within a society that no one questions them; they are also frequently accepted as the truth, and even as virtuous. Unfortunately, in medicine, our cultural beliefs include perfectionism, complete autonomy, overwork, and self-sacrifice (Shanafelt et al. 2019). In a survey of Australian and New Zealand veterinarians, a vast majority (88%) agreed that fatigue was inevitable in the profession, and 72% said that burnout is a normal part of the job. Within that same group, 80% believed they should be at work even if they were showing signs of the flu, with not wanting to burden others as the primary reason. This particular data point is even more troubling given that it was collected during a global pandemic where the primary symptoms of the disease were similar to the flu (Connolly et al. 2022). This impulse to drive oneself to the point of exhaustion, ignoring all signals from our body that it needs rest, sets the stage for a host of physical and mental health concerns.

Furthermore, these entrenched cultural beliefs unfortunately influence attitudes toward seeking help. In a study examining the barriers to accessing mental health support amongst veterinary students in the United States, a prevalent belief emerged that veterinary school is inherently challenging, leading students to expect to feel miserable, overworked, and overwhelmed as par for the course. When misery is expected, experiencing it hardly seems abnormal. Consequently, 61% of these students expressed the belief that their struggles weren't severe enough to warrant seeking help (Hancock and karaffa 2022). Like the fable of the frog in slowly boiling water, these students became accustomed to suffering and even anticipated it, ultimately to their own detriment. Even when they recognized they were suffering, feelings of shame prevailed, as these students expressed that they shouldn't need help but should be able to fix their own problems (Hancock and Karaffa 2022).

Thankfully, culture can be shifted and changed. In recent years, there has been an increasing focus on mental health in the veterinary profession. The cultural shift is ongoing and not complete, as we still consistently see overwork and work–life conflict as significant stressors in the field (Andela 2020). However, there are signs of improvement. In sequential Merck Veterinary Wellbeing studies from 2019 to 2023, there has been increasing recognition that mental health care helps veterinarians lead healthier lives. We have also witnessed greater comfort in discussing mental health topics (Merck Animal Health 2023). Perhaps most promising, the number of veterinarians seeking mental health care has increased from 13% in 2017 to 23% in 2023 (Merck Animal Health 2023).

ACCESSIBILITY

There can be both practical and logistical barriers to mental health care. In one survey, 58.1% of Australian and New Zealand veterinarians reported experiencing difficulty obtaining time off work due to mental health concerns, 57.4% struggled with scheduling related care appointments, and 52.2% expressed concerns about the costs involved (Connolly et al. 2022). Each of these hurdles can deter individuals from seeking the help they need.

The emergence of telehealth services presents a promising solution to some of these obstacles. During the pandemic, legal regulations on telehealth were expanded, enabling greater access to a range of mental health services. Both synchronous and asynchronous telehealth platforms offer individuals greater flexibility and convenience in accessing therapy, circumventing issues related to scheduling conflicts and obtaining time off work. In asynchronous care, patients utilize a private chat for discussion with their mental health professional, while in synchronous care, video or voice calls are used to engage. Telehealth platforms, particularly asynchronous ones, can also be more affordable than in-person visits.

Healthcare benefits can also help with the affordability of treatment. In a recent survey of US veterinary professionals, 53% of veterinarians and 56% of support staff reported having health insurance that covers mental health treatment. Interestingly, 38% of vets and 37% of support staff were unsure whether their health insurance covered mental health, so the number of individuals with coverage may actually be higher (Volk et al. 2022). Certainly, an early action step in obtaining care is to check and understand your benefit coverage.

Veterinary professionals can also leverage resources such as employee assistance programs (EAPs) to overcome barriers to obtaining mental health care. EAPs are employer-sponsored programs designed to assist employees with personal matters, including mental health concerns, child and elder care, financial counseling, and legal issues. These programs often offer both confidential counseling services and referrals to therapists. However, while 31% of veterinarians and 36% of support staff report having access to an EAP, a notable 26% of veterinarians and 32% of support staff remain uncertain about its availability, suggesting a need for improved communication and awareness among veterinary professionals regarding these valuable resources (Volk et al. 2022).

For those without mental health benefits, low-cost mental health services such as sliding fee scales and community clinics offer accessible options for seeking support. When offered, sliding fee scales allow individuals to pay based on their income, reducing the financial burden of therapy sessions. Community clinics, often operated by nonprofit organizations, government agencies, or academic institutions, provide counseling (typically shorter-term, goal-oriented, and addressing specific life challenges), therapy (longer-term, more exploratory, and treating mental health disorders), and support groups at reduced rates or even free of charge. These affordable options help ensure that financial barriers do not completely prevent people from getting the help they need. That being said, veterinary professionals should be mindful that mental health care teams, like veterinary teams, also deserve fair compensation for their expertise and support. Both fields understand and sympathize with the difficult intersection between healthcare and cost.

In terms of obstacles, finding an in-person practitioner who accepts your benefits, or is otherwise affordable, and is accepting new clients can also be a challenge. Thankfully, there are also effective resources to help with this. One option is to reach out to your healthcare benefits team for assistance in locating in-network therapists or counselors covered by your insurance plan. Alternatively, veterinary professionals can turn to online search platforms, such as Psychology Today's website (psychologytoday.com), which hosts a vast database of mental health professionals. You can then search based on a variety of criteria, such as location, specialties, and services offered.

THE SPECTRUM OF MENTAL HEALTH CARE

In addressing mental health concerns, there is currently a spectrum of options available for support and treatment. Table 4.1 outlines the various types of professionals who provide mental health support and treatment, along with their qualifications.

Table 4.1 Mental health professionals.

Mental health professional	Degrees/licenses required	Services provided
Support groups	None	Peer support, sharing experiences, coping strategies, mutual understanding, community-building
Peer support	Lived experience, certification may be required for certain organizations	Sharing lived experiences, providing empathy and understanding, offering practical advice and coping skills
Counselor	Bachelor's or Master's degree in counseling or related field; licensure varies by state	Counseling individuals or groups, providing therapy for various mental health concerns, offering guidance and support
Pastors/priests	Ordination or religious education, some may have additional training in pastoral counseling	Spiritual guidance, counseling, offering emotional support and encouragement, providing prayer and religious rituals
Life coach	Certification from an accredited coaching program, may have Bachelor's or Master's degree in related field	Helping individuals set and achieve personal or professional goals, providing motivation, offering guidance and support
LMFT (licensed marriage and family therapist)	Master's degree in Marriage and Family Therapy, completion of supervised clinical experience, licensure	Counseling individuals, couples, and families, addressing relationship issues, providing therapy for mental health concerns within the context of relationships
MSW (social worker)	Master's degree in Social Work, completion of supervised clinical experoence, licensure	

(*Continued*)

Table 4.1 (Continued)

Mental health professional	Degrees/licenses required	Services provided
Psychologist	Ph.D. or Psy.D. in Psychology, completion of supervised clinical internship and postdoc, licensure	Assessing and diagnosing mental health disorders, providing therapy and counseling, conducting psychological evaluations, research
Psychiatrist	Medical degree (M.D. or D.O.), completion of residency in psychiatry, licensure	Diagnosing mental health disorders, prescribing medication, providing therapy and counseling, managing complex mental health cases
Pet loss grief counselor	Certification from an accredited program	Assisting individuals in Pet loss grief counselors play a crucial role in helping individuals navigate the often profound and complex emotions associated with the loss of a beloved animal companion. These professionals provide a safe and empathetic space for people to express their grief, validate their feelings, and offer coping strategies for pet loss.

There are two primary types of treatment for mental health conditions: psychotherapy and medication. In the following section, we will provide an overview of these therapies to help you become an informed patient who can advocate for your needs.

Much of the following discussion focuses on depression, as it is a common concern in veterinary medicine. This in no way means to imply that treatment of mental health concerns is limited to depression, but rather a structure to provide illustrative data around mental health treatment concisely. A complete discussion of the treatment of all mental health disorders is beyond the scope of this text.

PSYCHOTHERAPY

Psychotherapy, also known as talk therapy, involves a therapeutic relationship between a trained professional and an individual, couple, family, or group.

While the objectives of therapy can vary depending on the needs and circumstances of the patient(s), they often include improving overall mental well-being, establishing a sustainable work–life balance, facilitating behavior change, enhancing communication, strengthening personal and professional relationships, and developing effective coping skills.

There are a variety of therapeutic techniques and principles within the field of psychotherapy. The majority of practitioners use a blend of modalities based on their patients' needs and their personal preferences, training, and experience. For example, cognitive behavioral therapy (CBT) is a common set of techniques based on the principles that psychological distress arises from unhelpful thought patterns and behaviors, which can be relieved through cognitive restructuring and behavioral modification. Indeed, CBT is an evidence-based practice that has been shown across a myriad of studies to be beneficial in a wide variety of disorders and conditions of distress, specifically including improvement of depression, anxiety, and suicidal ideation in veterinary students (Hofmann et al. 2012; Melnyk et al. 2022). Table 4.2 provides examples of some common forms of psychotherapy.

Table 4.2 Types of pyschotherapy.

Psychotherapy encompasses a variety of therapeutic modalities, each with its unique approach and coping skills to help individuals overcome mental health concerns. These modalities can be adapted to the specific needs of individuals, and therapists often integrate multiple approaches to offer comprehensive care. The choice of therapy depends on the individual's diagnosis and preferences, and the therapist's expertise and training.

Below is a summary of common therapeutic modalities:

Cognitive Behavioral Therapy (CBT)

- **Focus**: Thoughts, feelings, and behaviors.
- **Key Components**: CBT aims to identify and challenge negative or distorted thought patterns and replace them with healthier, more realistic, and balanced thoughts. The premise is that thoughts influence emotions and behaviors, so adapting the way one thinks can change the way one feels and acts.
- **Frequently utilized for**: Depression, anxiety, phobias, PTSD, and obsessive-compulsive disorder (OCD).

Dialectical Behavior Therapy (DBT)

- **Focus**: Emotional regulation and interpersonal effectiveness.
- **Key Components**: A form of CBT designed to help people manage intense emotions. DBT emphasizes mindfulness, acceptance of situations, and implementing effective change strategies. To do this, DBT emphasizes learning and practicing coping skills for distress tolerance, emotional regulation, and improving relationships through interpersonal effectiveness.
- **Frequently utilized for**: Borderline personality disorder (BPD), self-harm, suicidal behaviors, and eating disorders.

Psychodynamic Therapy

- **Focus**: Unconscious processes and early-life experiences.
- **Key Components**: Rooted in Freudian theory, psychodynamic therapy explores how unconscious conflicts and past experiences (especially in one's childhood) shape present behavior. It emphasizes insight into these unconscious processes as a way to resolve psychological distress.
- **Frequently utilized for**: Depression, anxiety, and complex mental health disorders.

Humanistic Therapy

- **Focus**: Personal growth and self-actualization.
- **Key Components**: Humanistic therapies, like **Client-Centered Therapy** (Carl Rogers) or **Gestalt Therapy** (Fritz Perls), emphasize personal responsibility, free will, and the innate human drive and desire for self-improvement. They focus on providing a nonjudgmental, empathetic environment to help individuals reach their full potential.
- **Frequently utilized for**: Self-esteem issues, relationship difficulties, and existential crises.

Family and Couples Therapy

- **Focus**: Interpersonal relationships within families or couples.
- **Key Components**: This modality examines the dynamics of relationships rather than focusing on individual issues. It seeks to improve communication, resolve conflicts, and strengthen emotional bonds. **Structural Family Therapy** and **Emotionally Focused Therapy** are examples.
- **Frequently utilized for**: Marital problems, family conflicts, and parenting issues.

Mindfulness-based Therapies

- **Focus**: Mindfulness and present-moment awareness.
- **Key Components**: Therapies like **Mindfulness-Based Cognitive Therapy (MBCT)** combine mindfulness practices (awareness, acceptance, and staying present) with cognitive techniques to help individuals better manage stress, as well as symptoms of depression and anxiety.
- **Frequently utilized for**: Depression relapse prevention, stress reduction, and anxiety management.

(Continued)

Table 4.2 (Continued)

Prolonged Exposure Therapy (PE)

- **Focus**: Trauma processing.
- **Key Components:** PE helps individuals confront and process trauma-related thoughts, emotions, and situations in a controlled and systematic way. The main objective is to reduce trauma-induced symptoms by gradually decreasing the power and emotional charge of traumatic triggers. By consistently engaging in exposure exercises, the client's fear responses diminish, and they learn to cope with trauma-related memories and similar situations more effectively, reducing PTSD symptoms over time.
- **Frequently utilized for:** PTSD, trauma-related distress.

Eye Movement Desensitization and Reprocessing (EMDR)

- **Focus**: Trauma processing.
- **Key Components**: EMDR uses bilateral stimulation (eye movements or taps) while the individual recalls distressing events, helping them process traumatic memories in a less distressing way. The technique integrates components of cognitive-behavioral therapy and body-based techniques.
- **Frequently utilized for**: PTSD, trauma, and complex grief.

Acceptance and Commitment Therapy (ACT)

- **Focus**: Psychological flexibility and values-based living.
- **Key Components**: ACT encourages individuals to accept their thoughts and feelings rather than trying to eliminate, control, or push them away. The focus is on living a meaningful life based on the integration of personal values, while acknowledging the presence of painful thoughts or emotions.
- **Frequently utilized for**: Anxiety, depression, chronic pain, and stress.

Interpersonal Therapy (IPT)

- **Focus**: Interpersonal relationships and social roles.
- **Key Components**: IPT focuses on resolving interpersonal problems and improving social functioning to reduce psychological symptoms. It is structured and time-limited, typically lasting 12–16 weeks.
- **Frequently utilized for**: Depression, grief, and interpersonal disputes.

Solution-focused Brief Therapy (SFBT)

- **Focus**: Solutions and future goals.
- **Key Components**: SFBT is a short-term therapy that emphasizes finding solutions to current problems rather than exploring their causes. The focus is on building strengths, setting goals, and working toward a preferred future.
- **Frequently utilized for**: Short-term problems, goal achievement, and solution-building.

Symptoms of mental health disorders usually last at least several weeks and are pervasive throughout many contexts in one's life. If you question whether or not you may have a mental health condition, please seek the advice of a professional assessment in lieu of self-diagnosis.
References: DSM-V, Mayoclinic.org

Furthermore, it is worth noting that a successful therapeutic outcome is not determined solely by the psychological techniques used, but rather by a myriad of factors. For instance, the rapport built with your therapist, the amount of time spent engaged in sessions, and the frequency of mental health care have all demonstrated a positive impact on outcome (Bruijniks et al. 2020; Nordmo et al. 2020).

Later in this chapter, we will discuss other crucial factors for maximizing therapeutic success, including how to find the right therapist for you and ensure you and your therapist are on the same page regarding your goals and progress.

MEDICATION

Psychiatric medications, including antidepressants, antipsychotics, mood stabilizers, and anxiolytics, can be prescribed by physicians to help alleviate symptoms of mental illness.

These medications have been shown repeatedly to be of benefit in mental health treatment. Selective serotonin reuptake inhibitors (SSRIs), a common class of antidepressants, have a mean response rate of 51% in the treatment of depression (Leichsenring et al. 2022). However, we must acknowledge that a 51% response rate means that 49% of people did not respond. Why is that? Reasons for treatment failure are multifactorial. Broadly speaking, depression is a complex constellation of symptoms with biological, social, and psychological risk factors. Although medication can address biological factors, which for some patients may be enough to result in full symptom relief, it cannot fully address other aspects that may be contributing to one's depressive symptoms.

It should be noted that treatment adherence plays a significant role in symptom improvement. A meta-analysis found that 49% of patients on psychiatric medication are not adherent to their medication schedule (Semahegn et al. 2020). Indeed, people have a variety of reasons for not taking medications; those described in the literature include stigma, attitudes toward medications, side effects, treatment durations, difficulties navigating the healthcare system, cost of medications, and concerns about efficacy. In some cases, these concerns about efficacy may stem from inadequate patient education. Many of these medications take time to be effective, often a minimum of four to six weeks; 28% of patients in one study stopped taking their medications within a month (Jung et al. 2016). Furthermore, 63.1% of those patients did so without consulting their physician (Woo-Young 2016). This is particularly worrisome because consultation with one's physician may lead to an adjusted strategy that provides greater relief. In another study, 25% of people benefited from adding a second medication, and 50% improved when a different medication was tried (Connolly and Thase 2011).

There is room for education on both sides of the exam table on this issue. A substantial number of people receive their psychiatric medications from their primary care doctor. While this is certainly convenient and an excellent way for many people to access care quickly, a primary care doctor is not likely to have extensive training in diagnosing psychiatric illness, nor be as familiar with the wide variety of drugs and treatment protocols as a psychiatrist who specializes in the field. For example, just within the antidepressant category alone, there are seven different classes of medications with multiple drugs in each class (FDA 2019). A general physician's unfamiliarity with diagnostic and/or treatment protocols may lead to less-than-ideal treatment and results. Indeed, in one analysis of antidepressant use, 41% of medications were being underdosed (Davidson et al. 2020). If an initial treatment plan is not successful, consultation with a psychiatrist who specializes in the use of these medications is highly recommended.

Underlying all of these concerns is a common theme that psychiatric medication is not a "one and done" phenomenon for a significant portion of patients. There is often a period when medications are tried and sometimes replaced due to efficacy concerns, side effects, etc. This can be frustrating for the person seeking care, but, as the veterinarian in Story 4.1 expressed, seeing the process through can be well worth the effort. It is also worth considering that a combination of different antidepressant medications may yield better results than antidepressant monotherapy, as illustrated by a recent meta-analysis (Henssler et al. 2022).

While the pharmacology and application of these medications are beyond the scope of this discussion, some of them are also employed in veterinary medicine and, therefore, may be familiar. Be that as it may, it's important to remember that self-treatment is both illegal and unwise. Applications, dosages, and side effects can affect humans and animals differently, and prescription medication should be monitored by a physician. Just as you would not want a human medical practitioner prescribing for their animal, veterinarians should not prescribe for themselves.

STORY 4.1 PSYCHIATRIC MEDICATION

My journey with psychiatric medication was a long, twisted road that was not entirely pleasant. My general practitioner (GP) prescribed my first one for me in my twenties. The medication was Prozac, and it worked in a way. I was no longer suicidal. I didn't even really feel depressed, but I was also just flat. The other side effects, like weight gain and loss of libido, were also not pleasant. I tried a second one at some point; another SSRI, Zoloft, and the results were similar.

It made me really hesitant to take medication. For instance, even though I have pretty bad insomnia, I was super resistant to taking anything for it. I felt like I shouldn't need it, that my problems at that point weren't "bad enough" to warrant it, and the previous side effects made me super leery of trying anything. I had a couple of serious bouts of depression in vet school and my residency that I just sort of white-knuckled through, in part due to that previous experience.

I was diagnosed in my 40s with ADHD, and I had finally found a psychiatrist who I clicked with. We started working with ADHD meds, which, after a bit of trial and error, were helping me a great deal. Then the pandemic hit and everything just got harder. I was really struggling. I will never forget that we were talking about my sleep, or lack thereof, and I had once again been hesitant about medications. She actually got mad at me. She snapped at me. "You have to sleep! I know you are worried about the meds, and if you get addicted, we will deal with that later, but right now you need rest!"

Her frustration broke through my stubbornness. I recognized that feeling as a clinician, when you have a solution but the client just won't do it and you can see they are struggling and it's just so unnecessary. And the meds worked. Up until then, I don't think I had slept more than four hours at a time my whole life, and all the sudden I was getting at least seven hours a night.

I'm so glad I took that step, because about a year later, my marriage started falling apart and my depression came roaring back. She is a really good doctor. She knew to ask the hard question, and unfortunately, the answer was yes. I was suicidal. It was mild, but it was there. I had "toughed it out" until I was in real trouble. She started talking about medication. I was ready for it to be just like my past experiences, but I accepted that dull was better than dead. She listened to me about the last medication experience and ran a genetic screen that showed, indeed, I had a gene linked to increased side effects with SSRIs. She chose a different medication class, and the result was so much better than I had hoped for. No real side effects. I was myself. I was just in control in a way I don't think I ever had been. I'm really grateful that she was able to break through my hesitation, because I know that it helped pull me out of a really dark time, and I now feel better than I ever have. The only frustration I have is that I didn't find this medication 20 years ago.

BENEFITS OF COMBINED CARE

The use of psychotherapy and medication is not mutually exclusive; in fact, numerous studies have shown that they are best utilized in concert. In an umbrella review of meta-analyses, both psychotherapy and psychiatric medication showed benefits over placebo, while a combination of the two showed a moderate effect size benefit over either treatment individually (Leichsenring et al. 2022).

Additional well-being interventions have also been shown to have a favorable impact on psychological health, underlying the shift in nomenclature from mental illness to mental health. Our psychological health does not exist in a vacuum, and healthy activities such as sleep, nutrition, mindfulness, and exercise can have a profound impact on mental health conditions. The addition of these self-care techniques can amplify the outcomes of the traditional therapies discussed above (Grajek et al. 2022; Henriksson et al. 2022; Scott et al. 2021). It is also well-established that the health of your social relationships has a profound impact on your mental health (Wickramaratne et al. 2022). As tempting as it might be to put your relationships on the back burner when you get busy, you do so at your own peril.

It must be stated that the exact treatment formula that works will vary from person to person. However, what is shared is the importance of having a plan. Knowing that exercise and therapy help our mental health is a solid start, but unless those activities are scheduled and actually engaged in, they remain just concepts. The Merck Veterinary Wellbeing study confirmed in 2023 that a stress management plan was an essential protective factor in well-being for both veterinarians and support staff (Volk et al. 2022).

ADVANCED THERAPIES AND THE FUTURE

Despite the benefits of care, response is not universal. For instance, over 12 months, an estimated 8.9 million people will be on medication for major depressive disorder; approximately one-third of them will be treatment resistant, meaning they do not show improvement after treatment trials with two medications (Zhdanava et al. 2021). Thankfully, the spectrum of care does not end with psychotherapy, well-being interventions, and conventional medications.

There are emerging innovative therapies, such as transcranial magnetic stimulation (TMS), which show significant improvements in major depressive disorder and treatment-resistant depression in 28 out of 29 studies in one meta-analysis (De Risio et al. 2020). Additionally, there are recent advancements using ketamine therapy, which have shown promising improvements in response rates, and even remission in the treatment of various psychiatric disorders, including treatment-resistant depression and posttraumatic stress disorder (PTSD; Alnefeesi et al. 2022; Feder et al. 2021).

Further new treatments may also be on the horizon, with ongoing clinical trials exploring the therapeutic potential of various psychedelic substances such as lysergic acid diethylamide (LSD), methylenedioxymethamphetamine (MDMA), psilocybin, and ayahuasca. Despite their current classification as illegal recreational drugs, preliminary findings in clinical settings suggest positive outcomes, which could shift their legal status (Luoma et al. 2020).

MAXIMIZING SUCCESS

MATCHING WITH THE RIGHT PRACTITIONER

Sir William Osler, often called the father of modern medicine, is frequently credited with saying, "It is sometimes more important to know what sort of patient has a disease than what sort of disease a patient has" (Elpern 2021). An experienced clinician will tell you that for a therapy to be successful, tailoring to the patient is required. While it's important to consider scientifically validated success rates in any medical therapy, they mean nothing if a patient cannot or will not participate in that therapy. Psychotherapy is no exception. Certainly, a patient's instincts about what care they need may not be completely correct. Still, as one author stated, the most successful therapeutic relationships will "adapt psychotherapy to the particulars of the individual patient but do so according to generalities identified by research" (Norcross and Wampold 2011).

Table 4.3 reviews various aspects of therapy that can contribute to a "good fit" between those seeking help and their mental health practitioners. The contribution of these individual aspects to overall success is still a matter of debate, but receiving preferred therapy has been shown to improve clinical outcomes and significantly reduce dropout rates (Cooper and Norcross 2016). Similar to our recommendations for medication, if you don't have a good fit with your therapist the first time around, don't give up. It may take a couple of tries before you find a therapist who is a good match for your needs and preferences. In Story 4.2, a practice manager discusses why her current therapist is a good match for her.

Table 4.3 Matching with a therapist.

Questions one may want to ask when finding a therapist:
• When you heard about the things I want to address in therapy, do those feel within your area of expertise to help me with?
• Have you worked with other clients in the veterinary medicine field or other healthcare professions?
• What is your experience working with clients where (sexual orientation, cultural identity, religion/spirituality, etc.) is an important part of their identity and is a desired area of focus in therapy?
• I have heard that therapists have different approaches to how they provide psychotherapy. Can you tell me the styles of therapy you use to help clients?
• I have heard that therapists can vary in terms of how much feedback they give to clients. Can you tell me about your style here?
• How do we assess if therapy is working effectively?
• I have heard that therapists can vary in terms of how much they provide support during sessions, compared to giving direction to their clients. Can you tell me about your style here?
• I also heard that therapists can vary in terms of how much they tend to set goals for clients between sessions (e.g. homework). Can you tell me what you tend to do?
• How do you like to get feedback if there is something about our therapy work together that isn't sitting right with me?
• Do you accept my insurance? If not, do you provide documentation to help me submit for partial reimbursement for service fees to my insurance provider?
• Do you offer a sliding-scale pay structure in certain circumstances for clients?

STORY 4.2 THERAPY MATCH

I love my therapist for so many reasons. First, she worked with a veterinary social worker. This has given her some important insight into the struggles in a veterinary hospital and the pressures of practice management. It's super helpful to have someone understand the pressures you are actually discussing with them. I also enjoy working with her because she does give me homework or finds ways to challenge me to push myself a little bit. Validation is great, but I recently joined therapy because I wanted to get into the nitty-gritty of why I am the way I am and actions to improve my life. She pushes me. No topic is off limits. I adore my therapist and I've grown so much since working with her.

It's important to ask for a clinician's credentials and licensure, and they will expect this. Licensed mental health professionals are governed by a board in their state, for example, the California Board of Psychology, which also keeps you protected should you reach out to them for assistance or to file a complaint. Furthermore, while "psychologist" and "psychiatrist" are legally protected terms indicating advanced education, clinical experience, and passing board examinations, "counselor" and "therapist" are not. There are a variety of unlicensed counselors, such as life coaches and grief counselors, with varying levels of training. It is absolutely appropriate to ask your clinician what degree(s) they hold, where they went to graduate or medical school, their approaches to therapy, the populations they work with, their areas of expertise, their fees, cancellation policies, availability, and which states they are licensed in. Table 4.4 provides a summary of mental health professionals, their roles, education, and licensure.

Table 4.4 Mental health professionals.

There are several different types of mental health professionals, each with specialized training, roles, and approaches to helping individuals with emotional, psychological, or psychiatric concerns.

Below is a summary of common mental health professions and what they focus on:

Psychiatrist (MD or DO)

- **Role**: Medical doctor specializing in mental health, including diagnosis, treatment, and prevention of mental, emotional, and behavioral disorders.
- **Focus**: Biological aspects of mental health conditions.
- **What They Do**: Psychiatrists can prescribe medications (like antidepressants, mood stabilizers, or antipsychotics), offer psychotherapy, and conduct medical evaluations. They often manage severe mental illnesses like schizophrenia, bipolar disorder, and major depressive disorder.
- **Training**: Medical degree (MD or DO) followed by a residency in psychiatry.

Licensed Psychologist (PhD or PsyD)

- **Role**: Doctorate-level mental health professional specializing in testing, diagnosing, and treating psychological disorders through various forms of psychotherapy.
- **Focus**: Cognitive, emotional, and behavioral aspects of mental health.
- **What They Do**: Licensed psychologists test, assess, and treat mental health issues using evidence-based psychotherapies and manualized treatment interventions. They cannot prescribe medications in most jurisdictions (except in some states in the United States where specially trained psychologists can).
- **Training**: Doctorate degree in psychology (PhD or PsyD) with supervised clinical experience.

Licensed Professional Counselor (LPC)/Licensed Mental Health Counselor (LMHC)

- **Role**: Licensed counselors help people gain personal insights, develop strategies, and enact real-world solutions to the problems and challenges they face across all facets of life.
- **Focus**: Mental, behavioral, and emotional problems and disorders.
- **What They Do**: LPCs/LMHCs work with people across the lifespan and address issues related to life transitions, academic and career concerns, and challenging situations such as a chronic illness or disruptive event. As trained and credentialed professionals, they aim to understand and have sensitivity to the effects of diverse individual, familial, and cultural factors.
- **Training**: Master's degree in counseling or a related field, with supervised clinical hours and state licensure.

Marriage and Family Therapist (MFT)

- **Role**: Therapist focusing on interpersonal dynamics within families and couples.
- **Focus**: Relationship issues, family dynamics, and interpersonal communication.
- **What They Do**: MFTs specialize in helping couples and families address issues like marital conflict, parenting challenges, or family trauma. They work to improve communication and resolve conflicts within relationships.
- **Training**: Master's degree in marriage and family therapy, with clinical supervision and state licensure.

Clinical Social Worker (LCSW)

- **Role**: Social worker trained to provide psychotherapy and support services.
- **Focus**: Addressing both emotional and social/environmental factors affecting mental health.
- **What They Do**: LCSWs offer therapy to individuals, families, and groups, while also addressing social issues like long-term treatment planning, housing, employment, or access to resources, benefits, and services. They work with diverse populations, including those facing poverty, trauma, or substance abuse.
- **Training**: Master's degree in social work (MSW) with a focus on clinical practice, plus supervised hours for licensure.

(*Continued*)

Table 4.4 (Continued)

Psychiatric Nurse Practitioner (PMHNP)

- **Role**: Advanced practice nurse with specialized training in mental health care.
- **Focus**: Holistic care, often blending medication management and psychotherapy.
- **What They Do**: PMHNPs can diagnose mental health disorders, prescribe medications, and provide psychotherapy. They work with individuals across the lifespan, addressing mental health needs in both clinical and community settings.
- **Training**: Master's or doctoral degree in nursing with a psychiatric/mental health specialization, and national certification.

Substance Abuse Counselor/Addiction Counselor

- **Role**: Counselor specializing in the treatment of individuals with substance-use disorders.
- **Focus**: Substance abuse, addiction recovery, and relapse prevention.
- **What They Do**: These counselors help individuals struggling with drug or alcohol addiction through counseling, treatment plans, and support groups. They often work in rehab centers, community health organizations, or private practice.
- **Training**: Varies by state and organization but typically involves a bachelor's or master's degree in counseling or a related field, plus certification or licensure.

Pastoral Counselor

- **Role**: Counselor integrating psychological counseling with spiritual guidance.
- **Focus**: Mental health within the context of religious or spiritual beliefs.
- **What They Do**: Pastoral counselors offer therapy that incorporates religious or spiritual perspectives, often helping individuals navigate emotional challenges through their faith. They may work in religious organizations, hospitals, or private practice.
- **Training**: Master's degree in counseling or divinity, with specialized training in pastoral care and counseling.

Each of these professions brings a unique approach to mental health care, and individuals often work collaboratively across disciplines to provide comprehensive support tailored to each person's needs.

CONTINUED SUCCESS

Preferences should be an ongoing conversation throughout therapy, even beginning before your first session as most clinicians offer consult calls free of charge. For many people, boundaries can be a helpful place to start. There may be certain topics you are not ready to discuss, or don't want to discuss at all. For example, a mental health professional may start discussing their own pets as a well-intentioned attempt to build rapport. Despite these good intentions, this can feel violating and inappropriate to many veterinary professionals. It's perfectly reasonable to ask that they refrain from discussing their personal pets. Remember, this is your time as the person seeking treatment. If something isn't helpful or feels harmful, it's important to say so. Similarly, your mental health professional may suggest an exercise that you don't connect with. While it's certainly reasonable to give it a try, if you don't find it useful, discussing why is an important part of the therapeutic relationship; your practitioner should be open to this conversation. In an ideal scenario, your mental health professional will specifically and routinely solicit feedback on how things are feeling for you (Table 4.4).

Preferences should also include the incorporation of self-directed goals. What do you, the patient, want to get from this therapy? Is there a particular topic that you would like to discuss during the session? Are you looking for coping skills to better manage ongoing stress? Do you want to unpack some past experiences and how they might be influencing your behavior now? Are you feeling depressed or anxious and want to address those feelings and the potential underlying causes? Your mental health professional should be open to discussions of these objectives and should check in on progress as you work together.

At the end of the day, mental health care should instill a sense of agency in the person seeking it, which is the ability to take responsibility for and control of one's actions. Agency involves the capability to be self-reflective and self-regulating, as well as the ability to be responsible for and capable of controlling one's own actions in day-to-day life (Yao et al. 2022).

REFERENCES

Alnefeesi, Y., Chen-Li, D., Krane, E. et al. (2022). Real-world effectiveness of ketamine in treatment-resistant depression: a systematic review & meta-analysis. *Journal of Psychiatric Research* 151: 693–709.

American Psychiatric Association (2022). *Diagnostic and Statistical Manual of Mental Disorders: DSM-5-TR*, 14. Washington, DC: American Psychiatric Publishing.

Andela, M. (2020). Burnout, somatic complaints, and suicidal ideations among veterinarians: development and validation of the Veterinarians Stressors Inventory. *Journal of Veterinary Behavior* 37: 48–55.

Balch, B. (2022). From mental illness to mental health, AAMC. https://www.aamc.org/news/mental-illness-mental-health (accessed 1 April 2024).

Bartram, D.J., Yadegarfar, G., and Baldwin, D.S. (2009). A cross-sectional study of mental health and well-being and their associations in the UK veterinary profession. *Social Psychiatry and Psychiatric Epidemiology* 44: 1075–1085.

Best, C.O., Perret, J.L., Hewson, J. et al. (2020). A survey of veterinarian mental health and resilience in Ontario, Canada. *The Canadian Veterinary Journal* 61 (2): 166.

Bruijniks, S.J., Lemmens, L.H., Hollon, S.D. et al. (2020). The effects of once-versus twice-weekly sessions on psychotherapy outcomes in depressed patients. *The British Journal of Psychiatry* 216 (4): 222–230.

Connolly, C.E., Norris, K., Dawkins, S., and Martin, A. (2022). Barriers to mental health help-seeking in veterinary professionals working in Australia and New Zealand: a preliminary cross-sectional analysis. *Frontiers in Veterinary Science* 9: 1051571.

Connolly, K.R. and Thase, M.E. (2011). If at first you don't succeed: a review of the evidence for antidepressant augmentation, combination and switching strategies. *Drugs* 71: 43–64.

Cooper, M. and Norcross, J.C. (2016). A brief, multidimensional measure of clients' therapy preferences: the Cooper-Norcross Inventory of Preferences (C-NIP). *International Journal of Clinical and Health Psychology* 16 (1): 87–98.

Cormier, O. and Seddon, J. (2024). Alcohol-related stigma within the UK veterinary profession. *Veterinary Record* 195 (9).

da Silva, C.R., Gomes, A.A.D., dos Santos-Doni, T.R. et al. (2023). Suicide in veterinary medicine: a literature review. *Veterinary World* 16 (6): 1266.

Davidson, S.K., Romaniuk, H., Chondros, P. et al. (2020). Antidepressant treatment for primary care patients with depressive symptoms: data from the diamond longitudinal cohort study. *Australian and New Zealand Journal of Psychiatry* 54 (4): 367–381.

De Risio, L., Borgi, M., Pettorruso, M. et al. (2020). Recovering from depression with repetitive transcranial magnetic stimulation (rTMS): a systematic review and meta-analysis of preclinical studies. *Translational Psychiatry* 10 (1): 393.

Dyrbye, L.N., West, C.P., Sinsky, C.A. et al. (2017). Medical licensure questions and physician reluctance to seek care for mental health conditions. In: *Mayo clinic proceedings*, vol. 92, No. 10, 1486–1493. Elsevier.

Elpern, D.J. (2021). Musings on Osler mis-quoted. *The Pharos (Summer 2021)*, p. 25.

FDA. (2019). Depression medicines. *U.S. Food and Drug Administration*, FDA. www.fda.gov/consumers/womens-health-topics/depression-medicines (Accessed 15 April 2026).

Feder, A., Costi, S., Rutter, S.B. et al. (2021). A randomized controlled trial of repeated ketamine administration for chronic posttraumatic stress disorder. *American Journal of Psychiatry* 178 (2): 193–202.

Geuijen, P.M., van den Broek, S.J., Dijkstra, B.A. et al. (2021). Success rates of monitoring for healthcare professionals with a substance use disorder: a meta-analysis. *Journal of Clinical Medicine* 10 (2): 264–295.

Grajek, M., Krupa-Kotara, K., Białek-Dratwa, A. et al. (2022). Nutrition and mental health: a review of current knowledge about the impact of diet on mental health. *Frontiers in Nutrition* 9: 943998.

Hancock, T.S. and Karaffa, K.M. (2022). "Obligated to keep things under control": sociocultural barriers to seeking mental health services among veterinary medical students. *Journal of Veterinary Medical Education* 49 (5): 662–677.

Harling, M., Strehmel, P., Schablon, A., and Nienhaus, A. (2009). Psychosocial stress, demoralization and the consumption of tobacco, alcohol and medical drugs by veterinarians. *Journal of Occupational Medicine and Toxicology* 4 (1): 4.

Henriksson, M., Wall, A., Nyberg, J. et al. (2022). Effects of exercise on symptoms of anxiety in primary care patients: a randomized controlled trial. *Journal of Affective Disorders* 297: 26–34.

Henssler, J., Alexander, D., Schwarzer, G. et al. (2022). Combining antidepressants vs antidepressant monotherapy for treatment of patients with acute depression: a systematic review and meta-analysis. *JAMA Psychiatry* 79 (4): 300–312.

Hofmann, S.G., Asnaani, A., Vonk, I.J. et al. (2012). The efficacy of cognitive behavioral therapy: a review of meta-analyses. *Cognitive Therapy and Research* 36: 427–440.

Jung, W.Y., Jang, S.H., Kim, S.G. et al. (2016). Times to discontinue antidepressants over 6 months in patients with major depressive disorder. *Psychiatry Investigation* 13 (4): 440.

Kassem, A.M., Witte, T.K., Nett, R.J., and Carter, K.K. (2019). Characteristics associated with negative attitudes toward mental illness among US veterinarians. *Journal of the American Veterinary Medical Association* 254 (8): 979–985.

Leichsenring, F., Steinert, C., Rabung, S., and Ioannidis, J.P. (2022). The efficacy of psychotherapies and pharmacotherapies for mental disorders in adults: an umbrella review and meta-analytic evaluation of recent meta-analyses. *World Psychiatry* 21 (1): 133–145.

Luoma, J.B., Chwyl, C., Bathje, G.J. et al. (2020). A meta-analysis of placebo-controlled trials of psychedelic-assisted therapy. *Journal of Psychoactive Drugs* 52 (4): 289–299.

Mason, D.S., Tenney, L., Hellyer, P.W., and Newman, L.S. (2018). Prescription opioid epidemic: do veterinarians have a dog in the fight? *American Journal of Public Health* 108 (9): 1162–1163.

Melnyk, B.M., Hoying, J., Hsieh, A.P. et al. (2022). Effects of a cognitive-behavioral skills building program on the mental health outcomes and healthy lifestyle behaviors of veterinary medicine students. *Journal of the American Veterinary Medical Association* 260 (7): 789–795.

Merck Animal Health. (2023). *Veterinary Wellbeing Presentation* [PowerPoint]. https://www.merck-animal-health-usa.com/offload-downloads/2023-vet-wellbeing-presentation (accessed 1 October 2025).

Michaelson, J., Mahony, S., and Schifferes, J. (2012). *Measuring Wellbeing: A Guide for Practitioners*. London: New Economics Foundation.

Miller, J.M. and Beaumont, J.J. (1995). Suicide, cancer, and other causes of death among California veterinarians, 1960-1992. *American Journal of Industrial Medicine* 27 (1): 37–49.

Mykyta, L. (2023). *Work Conditions and Serious Psychological Distress Among Working Adults Aged 18-64: United States, 2021*. US Department of Health and Human Services, Centers for Disease Control and Prevention, National Center for Health Statistics.

Nett, R.J., Witte, T.K., Holzbauer, S.M. et al. (2015). Risk factors for suicide, attitudes toward mental illness, and practice-related stressors among US veterinarians. *Journal of the American Veterinary Medical Association* 247 (8): 945–955.

Norcross, J.C. and Wampold, B.E. (2011) 'What works for whom: Tailoring psychotherapy to the person', Journal of Clinical Psychology, 67(2), pp. 127–132. https://doi.org/10.1002/jclp.20764. p. 131.

Nordmo, M.N., Sønderland, N.M., Havik, O.E. et al. (2020). Effectiveness of open-ended psychotherapy under clinically representative conditions. *Frontiers in Psychiatry* 11: 384.

Pohl, R., Botscharow, J., Böckelmann, I., and Thielmann, B. (2022). Stress and strain among veterinarians: a scoping review. *Irish Veterinary Journal* 75 (1): 15.

Schwerdtfeger, K.A., Bahramsoltani, M., Spangenberg, L. et al. (2020). Depression, suicidal ideation and suicide risk in German veterinarians compared with the general German population. *Veterinary Record* 186 (15): e2.

Scoresby, K., Jurney, C., Fackler, A. et al. (2023). Relationships between diversity demographics, psychological distress, and suicidal thinking in the veterinary profession: a nationwide cross-sectional study during COVID-19. *Frontiers in Veterinary Science 10.*

Scott, A.J., Webb, T.L., Martyn-St James, M. et al. (2021). Improving sleep quality leads to better mental health: a meta-analysis of randomised controlled trials. *Sleep Medicine Reviews* 60: 101556.

Semahegn, A., Torpey, K., Manu, A. et al. (2020). Psychotropic medication non-adherence and its associated factors among patients with major psychiatric disorders: a systematic review and meta-analysis. *Systematic Reviews* 9: 1–18.

Shanafelt, T.D., Schein, E., Minor, L.B. et al. (2019). Healing the professional culture of medicine. In: *Mayo Clinic Proceedings*, vol. 94, No. 8, 1556--1566. Elsevier.

Stein, D.J., Palk, A.C., and Kendler, K.S. (2021). What is a mental disorder? An exemplar-focused approach. *Psychological Medicine* 51 (6): 894–901.

Volk, J.O., Schimmack, U., Strand, E.B. et al. (2022). Executive summary of the Merck Animal Health Veterinarian Wellbeing Study III and Veterinary Support Staff Study. *Journal of the American Veterinary Medical Association* 260 (12): 1547–1553.

Wickramaratne, P.J., Yangchen, T., Lepow, L. et al. (2022). Social connectedness as a determinant of mental health: a scoping review. *PLoS One* 17 (10): e0275004.

Witte, T.K., Spitzer, E.G., Edwards, N. et al. (2019). Suicides and deaths of undetermined intent among veterinary professionals from 2003 through 2014. *Journal of the American Veterinary Medical Association* 255 (5): 595–608.

Yao, X., Dong, B., and Ji, W. (2022). Formulation and clients' agency in cognitive behavioral therapy. *Frontiers in Psychology* 13: 810437.

Zhdanava, M., Pilon, D., Ghelerter, I. et al. (2021). The prevalence and national burden of treatment-resistant depression and major depressive disorder in the United States. *The Journal of Clinical Psychiatry* 82 (2): 29169.

CHAPTER 5 Suicidality in Veterinary Medicine

Carrie Jurney, DVM, DACVIM (Neurology)[1] and Tracy Witte, PhD[2]

[1] *Not One More Vet, Inc., San Francisco, CA, USA*
[2] *Department of Psychological Sciences, Auburn University, Auburn, AL, USA*

INTRODUCTION

As we touched on in the previous chapter, unfortunately, veterinary professionals have consistently been shown to have elevated risk for suicidality. In an analysis of veterinary professionals who had died by suicide in the United States between 2003 and 2014, veterinarians, veterinary technicians, and technologists were determined to have higher suicide rates than the general population, whereas this was not true for veterinary assistants and laboratory animal caretakers (Witte et al. 2019). Unfortunately, this is not the only study to highlight this concern in the veterinary profession (e.g. Tomasi et al. 2019).

This chapter seeks to shed light on the prevalence, risk factors, and critical strategies for identification and intervention. By acknowledging these challenges and fostering a culture of support and mental health awareness, this chapter aims to equip veterinary professionals with the tools necessary to navigate this delicate terrain and promote a healthier, resilient veterinary community.

SPECTRUM OF SUICIDAL BEHAVIOR

Suicidality exists on a continuum. People are not simply 0% or 100% suicidal, and the concept includes several related but distinct components: suicide ideation, suicide attempts, and – tragically in some cases – death. Suicidal ideation refers to thoughts about death or killing oneself. These may be passive, such as "I wish I wouldn't wake up," or active, involving plans about method, timing, or location. Suicide attempts involve taking action with at least some intent to die, even if the behavior does not result in injury or require medical care. Finally, suicide deaths occur when self-inflicted behavior leads to a fatal outcome.

Nett et al. (2015) found that one in six veterinarians (16.67%) experience suicidal ideation during their careers – about 2.7 times the rate of the general population (approx 6–8%; Baca-García et al. 2008). Elevated rates have also been observed among other health care workers, including surgeons in the United States, Italy, and Sweden (14.9%, 18%, and 12%, respectively) (Shanafelt et al. 2011; Wall e al. 2014). Yet, the presence of ideation does not inevitably progress to action. Many people experiencing suicidal thoughts remain ambivalent about dying and are primarily seeking relief from overwhelming distress (Teismann et al. 2024).

In population research, roughly two-thirds of individuals with ideation never attempt suicide at all, and only about 7% attempt within two years of the onset of ideation (Nock et al. 2008; Have et al. 2009). Still, history matters: people with previous ideation or attempts are significantly more likely to attempt in the future, which is why any suicidal symptoms or history must be taken seriously (Daray et al., 2025). In veterinary contexts, there is additional concern that veterinarians appear more likely to die on their first attempt, likely related to access to and knowledge of highly lethal means (Nett et al., 2020). Lethality varies substantially by method, ranging from approximately 89.7% for firearms to 4% for cutting injuries (Cai et al. 2022). These topics are explored further in later sections on euthanasia and means safety.

CONTEMPORARY THEORIES OF SUICIDE

Many scientific frameworks try to explain why suicide happens. One of the most influential is the Interpersonal Theory of Suicide (IPTS), which proposes that suicidal thoughts develop when someone feels like a burden and disconnected from others. However, thoughts alone are not enough; a person must also have the capability to act, meaning reduced fear of death and greater tolerance for pain, often shaped through repeated exposure to distressing or painful experiences (Joiner, 2005; Van Orden et al., 2010).

Newer models build on this foundation. The ideation-to-action framework emphasizes that the causes of suicidal thoughts are not the same as the causes of suicide attempts, which helps explain why many people experience ideation, but far fewer make attempts (Klonsky et al., 2014). Klonsky and May's (2015) Three-Step Theory (3ST) describes a similar pathway: psychological pain and hopelessness generate suicidal ideation, which becomes stronger when pain outweighs connection, and attempts occur only with suicidal capability. 3ST clarifies that capability has three parts: dispositional (such as impulsivity), acquired (habituation to death), or practical (access to lethal means).

Other theories add further nuance. The Integrated Motivational–Volitional (IMV) model, for instance, describes how underlying factors (e.g. genetic, psychological, and life events) make an individual vulnerable to ideation (O'Connor, 2011). The presence of certain psychological states (defeat, humiliation, and entrapment) drives the emergence of ideation. Finally, there is a set of volitional moderators, which mediate the transition from ideation to attempt (i.e. impulsivity, acquired capability through things like self-harm or high-risk occupations, and history of or exposure to the suicidal behavior of others; O'Connor, 2011).

Across these theories, a consistent pattern emerges: psychological pain drives suicidal ideation, and capability determines whether someone attempts or dies by suicide. In veterinary medicine, this distinction helps shed light on specific risk factors inherent to the profession. The majority of veterinary professionals who engage in clinical work are exposed to death and, more specifically, euthanasia, which may contribute to acquired or practical capability. These issues are explored in later sections.

SUICIDALITY IN VETERINARY MEDICINE

Suicidality among veterinary professionals first appeared in research in the 1980s. Studies from the United States and the United Kingdom analyzing causes of death from the 1940s to the 1970s reported increased mortality ratios (the ratio of recorded vs expected deaths for that population) of 1.7 and 2.1, respectively (Blair and Hayes, 1982; Kinlen, 1983). Since then, elevated suicidality has been consistently documented in veterinary populations worldwide, including in Scotland, Wales, Norway, Germany, Finland, Australia, and Hong Kong (Bartram and Baldwin, 2010; da Silva et al. 2023; Chan 2023).

The persistent and widespread nature of this issue raises a critical question: *Why is this happening?* Suicidal behavior often stems from an interplay of circumstances, as well as risk and protective factors. In the veterinary profession, occupational stressors such as heavy workloads, financial debt, difficult client interactions, and performing euthanasia have been proposed as contributors to suicidality (da Silva et al., 2023).

At an individual level, mental health disorders – including anxiety and depression, which are more prevalent among veterinary professionals – also increase the risk of suicidality (Platt et al., 2012; Schunter et al., 2022). However, it is essential to recognize that veterinary professionals are more than their jobs. Their risk factors extend beyond their occupation, underscoring the need for a holistic exploration of the issue.

DEMOGRAPHIC TRENDS IN SUICIDALITY

Demographic patterns in suicidality among veterinary professionals mirror broader trends in veterinary mental health. Female veterinarians generally report a higher proportional risk of death than male veterinarians (Witte et al., 2019; Tomasi et al., 2019). However, interpreting these findings requires context from the general population, as men generally have a higher suicide rate than women. According to the WHO, the global age-standardized suicide rate is approximately 9 deaths per 100,000 people each year, with 12.6 per 100,000 for men and 5.4 per 100,000 for women (WHO, 2014).

This demographic risk is more pronounced in the United States, where men are roughly 3.7 times more likely to die by suicide than women, and this pattern persists among veterinarians (CDC, 2022; Witte et al., 2019; Tomasi, 2019). Yet, female veterinarians and veterinary technicians face a proportionally greater increase in risk than women in the general population. Put another way, although a male veterinarian might have a higher absolute risk for suicide compared to a female veterinarian (since men are generally more likely to die by suicide), a female veterinarian's occupation increases her risk for suicide more than a male veterinarian's occupation does. In a review of 11,620 veterinarian death records from 1979 to 2015, 398 deaths were attributed to suicide, 326 among men and 72 among women. Based on expected deaths in the general population, only 156 deaths would have been anticipated among men and 20 among women, indicating elevated mortality ratios for both. Importantly, the mortality ratio was higher among female veterinarians, underscoring disproportionate risk relative to women outside the profession (Tomasi 2019).

Sexual and gender minority groups also experience heightened suicidality both generally and in veterinary medicine. Transgender, nonbinary, and bisexual veterinary professionals report significantly higher rates of suicidal ideation (Scoresby et al., 2023). Among bisexual veterinarians, 39% report lifetime ideation, compared with 23% of gay or lesbian veterinarians and 13.9% of heterosexual colleagues. This pattern aligns closely with US population data: approximately 40% of bisexual adults report suicidal ideation, compared with 25% of gay or lesbian adults and 14% of heterosexual adults (CDC, 2022). Elevated risk may reflect lower perceived belonging and the compounded effects of stigma and discrimination (Salway et al., 2019).

Job type and role also influence suicide risk. Across multiple studies, companion animal, shelter medicine, and exotic animal medicine work with an increased risk of current or historical depression, serious psychological distress, and/or suicidality (Tomasi et al. 2019; Nett et al. 2015). In a large US survey, associate veterinarians had significantly higher rates of serious psychological distress than practice owners, and relief veterinarians reported the highest prevalence of depressive episodes, suicidal ideation, and prior suicide attempts of any practice role (Nett et al., 2015). However, the sample size of the relief population was small, and this did not reach statistical significance (Nett et al., 2015).

In what is, to our knowledge, the only study of suicide mortality among veterinary support staff, male veterinary technicians and technologists show a markedly higher mortality risk than male veterinarians, with mortality ratios of 5.0 compared with 1.6 (Witte et al., 2019). Interestingly, this was not observed for female veterinary technicians and technologists, whose standardized mortality ratio of 2.3 was nearly identical to that of female veterinarians (2.4).

Other studies have found a general increase in nonfatal suicidal behaviors in veterinary staff. In a sample of 2,208 veterinary professionals, veterinary technicians, unlicensed assistants, and customer service staff reported higher rates of suicidal ideation and planning than veterinarians (Scoresby et al., 2023). Similar trends appear in other fields: nonphysician healthcare workers often report higher suicidality than physicians (Olfson et al., 2023). Demographic differences, income disparities, workplace control, and occupational stressors likely contribute to this pattern and are discussed in Chapters 2, 3, 6, and 8.

EUTHANASIA AND SUICIDALITY

Many veterinary professionals do not view euthanasia as detrimental to their well-being, describing it instead as an act of compassion (Waitz-Kudla et al., 2023). Yet this normalization can obscure subtle psychological effects, especially among professionals already experiencing other stressors. The major contemporary theories of suicide help explain why this aspect of veterinary work may contribute to increased risk. As discussed earlier, many of the theories of suicide say that to progress from ideation requires acquiring suicidal capability. The 3ST adds greater context, defining capability as dispositional, acquired, or practical.

Within this framework, euthanasia has been discussed as a source of acquired and practical capability. Performing euthanasia requires overcoming the fear of causing death (acquired capability); discussing death as a solution to suffering (acquired capability); and practical knowledge about, as well as access to lethal drugs (practical capability).

ACQUIRED CAPABILITY

Fearlessness about death, a component of acquired capability, has been shown to be an independent predictor of suicide attempts and also has been related to attempt lethality (Ferm et al., 2020; Andreo-Jover et al., 2024). A 2013 study of veterinary students showed that experience with companion animal euthanasia, but not other medical procedures, was indirectly associated with fearlessness about death (Witte et al. 2013).

There is also evidence that exposure to euthanasia directly impacts veterinarians' feelings on both human euthanasia and suicide. In one study, veterinarians and the general population supported physician-assisted suicide at nearly identical rates (75% vs 73%). However, veterinarians more often cited minimizing suffering as a core reason for their support (Lerner et al. 2011). That reasoning mirrors the common clinical justification for animal euthanasia and can extend to beliefs about suicide. In a 2023 focus group study of practicing veterinarians, participants described how frequent discussions about the "kindness" of humane death made the idea of using pentobarbital for personal suicide seem more acceptable (Waitz-Kudla et al. 2023).

Frequency of exposure also seems to play a role. Veterinarians performing euthanasia five or more times per week reported significantly higher rates of serious suicidal ideation (Dalum et al. 2024). Recent surveys suggest that workloads of practicing veterinarians have increased in recent years, now approaching this threshold. A 2023 practice-level survey reported an average of 17 euthanasia procedures per month (4.25/week), which was an increase from the previous survey (Zakharankov 2023). As this average grows closer to the level associated with increased risk of suicidal ideation, this is a point of concern.

Although it has not been specifically studied in terms of suicidality, more morally objectionable forms of euthanasia, such as economic and convenience euthanasia, have been shown to contribute to adverse mental health outcomes such as psychological distress and burnout (Moses et al. 2018; Zakharankov 2023). To that point, shelter veterinarians, who experience a higher level of non-medically driven euthanasia, experience a higher rate of suicidal ideation than small animal practice veterinarians (30.4% vs 19.0%; Nett et al., 2015).

Among veterinary technicians and animal-care workers, euthanasia has been linked to negative well-being and mental health outcomes, especially when there is a strong attachment to animals or moral conflict about the decision (Hill et al., 2020; Kogan et al., 2020). However, these studies focus on mental health strain rather than suicidality outcomes, and further research is needed before drawing firm conclusions. It is common for technicians to assist with euthanasias and, in some cases, perform them, so their exposure level is likely similar to that of veterinarians. Furthermore, technicians often echo many of the same sentiments about euthanasia as a way to end suffering, which may in turn increase their risk for acquired capability.

PRACTICAL CAPABILITY

Aside from the psychological changes that can occur via repeated exposure and habituation to euthanasia, access to lethal means is another important concern. In the general population, access and familiarity with highly lethal methods significantly increase the likelihood that a suicide attempt will result in death. A systematic review found that people with occupational access to lethal means, such as medications or firearms, had higher suicide rates than those without such access (Milner et al., 2017). The act of euthanasia requires both knowledge of and access to lethal drugs such as pentobarbital. Unfortunately, this access and knowledge data bear out in veterinary populations, as pentobarbital poisoning is one of the most common, if not the most common, methods of suicide in veterinarians (Witte et al. 2019, Bartram and Baldwin 2010). The lethality of these medications likely contributes to the fact that veterinarians are more likely to die on their first attempt when compared with both the general population and other veterinary professionals (Witte et al., 2019; Nett al., 2020).

In contrast, suicide deaths among veterinary technicians and technologists more often involve opioid poisoning rather than pentobarbital (Witte 2019). Opioids are potentially lethal, particularly in high doses or in combination with other substances, but they are generally considered less lethal than pentobarbital. This difference in suicide methods may reflect differences in practical capability: technicians frequently administer opioids during patient care, while veterinarians are more often responsible for giving euthanasia medications and have more in-depth knowledge on how to enact death with pentobarbital.

Witte et al. (2019) showed that when pentobarbital deaths were removed from their sample of suicide decedents, mortality ratios among veterinarians were indistinguishable from those of the general population. In other words, the elevated mortality ratios seen in male and female veterinarians in their sample were seemingly accounted for by pentobarbital as a suicide method. The same pattern was not true for other veterinary professionals in the sample. Similarly, international research shows that when access to highly lethal methods is reduced, overall suicide deaths decline, even if other methods remain available (Yip et al., 2012, Hawton et al., 2013). These findings are particularly important in prevention, which is discussed in the next section.

SUICIDE PREVENTION AND INTERVENTION

When there are indications that a person may be experiencing suicidal thoughts, timely intervention can reduce the likelihood of harm. Support during suicidal crises spans a broad spectrum, from informal peer contact to hospitalization. Detailed intervention training is beyond the scope of this chapter, although several established programs provide education in brief suicide intervention, including the QPR (Question Persuade Refer) Institute (provided for free via the AVMA https://www.avma.org/resources-tools/wellbeing/qpr-suicide-prevention-training) and Emotional CPR (https://emotional-cpr.org).

The goal of early intervention is not necessarily to resolve a crisis entirely. Rather, the goal is to provide support until other resources, like professional mental health care, are available. Crisis intervention training is therefore not about turning a layperson into a mental health professional. Rather, it prepares people to step in during a critical moment. In this way, crisis intervention is similar to CPR (Cardiopulmonary Resuscitation): it can be life-saving, even when it does not fully address the underlying cause of the emergency. Its purpose is to create safety long enough for further care to occur. Much as is the case with CPR, a suicidal crisis can escalate quickly, necessitating rapid intervention. In a study of suicide attempt survivors, 57.7% reported that ideation and planning began on the same day as the attempt (Bryan et al. 2023).

RECOGNIZING WARNING SIGNS FOR SUICIDE

One of the most common myths about suicide is that it occurs without warning. In reality, most suicides and attempts are preceded by warning signs. Warning signs are dynamic risk factors indicating imminent risk for suicide that can be readily observed and used by the lay public (Rudd et al., 2006). As an example, male gender is a well-established distal risk factor for suicide; however, knowing that a friend of yours is male is not very useful in identifying whether he is suicidal and needs help right now. In contrast, the knowledge that a friend has recently lost his job and has started drinking heavily could raise alarm bells and prompt you to explore the situation further. A study of attempt survivors found that 75.2% had exhibited at least one warning sign before acting (Bader et al. 2021). Table 5.1 lists common warning signs for suicide.

Our emphasis on warning signs should not be taken to mean that more static factors cannot be useful when evaluating an individual's overall likelihood of making a suicide attempt. A prior suicide attempt increases risk almost 40-fold, particularly when attempts have occurred within the preceding two years (Prabhakar et al. 2020; Owens et al. 2002). As such, all else being equal, if a friend or colleague is exhibiting suicide warning signs in combination with a history of suicidal behavior, even more caution should be taken. This is because two of the strongest predictors of suicide are a history of attempts and the presence of current suicidal symptoms (Chu et al., 2015).

Despite the increase in risk associated with historical attempts, approximately half of individuals who die by suicide do so on their first attempt (Bostwick et al. 2016), and this percentage appears higher in veterinary medicine (Witte 2019). Risk assessment, therefore, considers not only the presence of suicidal thoughts but their intensity, frequency, and degree of planning. Passive statements such as, "I do not want to be here," suggest distress but convey less urgency than thoughts involving specific methods, times and/or locations (e.g. "I want to drive my car off the Golden Gate Bridge tonight."). Consideration of a plan typically includes assessing intent (whether the person believes they will act), timing, and access to means, with those who have high intent to act soon and easy access to means being at higher risk (Posner et al. 2011).

Table 5.1 Suicidal risk factors

Verbal/emotional cues	Behavioral	Situational
Finality ex. "I can't do this anymore"	Previous self harm, including prior attempts and non-suicidal self injury	Job or financial loss
Hopelessness ex. "Nothing works"	Increase in alcohol or drug Use	Loss of or conflict in relationships
Burdensomeness ex "Everyone would be better off without me"	Dramatic mood swings	Trauma or abuse
Loneliness or abandonment ex. "No one cares about me"	Agitation or irritability	Mental illness
Desperation ex. "I can live like this"	Severe weight loss	Serious illness, including chronic pain
Self-hatred ex. "I'm the worst veterinarian in the world"	Sleep disturbances	Recent loss by suicide in family or community
Expressions of rage "Everyone will regret how they've treated me"	Social withdrawal	Discrimination
Expressions of desperation "I'm at the end of my rope"	Impulse engagement in risky activities	Barriers to accessing health care
		Access to means

Source: Adapted from WHO (2014), Hendin et al. (2004) and Rudd (2006).

Despite the weight of all of these factors, suicide prevention is not about filling out a risk assessment checklist. Most importantly, it is about connecting with a person in distress in a humane way. People who are feeling suicidal often try to communicate those feelings before acting. In a meta-analysis of suicide deaths, 45% of individuals had communicated their intentions before the act (Pompili et al. 2016). By engaging in open, compassionate dialogue, we can create opportunities for intervention and potentially save lives.

EMPATHIC SUPPORT

Phrases like "I can't do this anymore," or "I can't live like this anymore," are commonly used to express frustration. However, they can also signal suicidal ideation. The most straightforward way to determine if someone is considering suicide is to ask directly. While this can feel uncomfortable, a conversation is far less harmful than the regret of silence after a tragedy, and Table 5.2 provides examples of supportive phrasing to ask about suicidal thoughts. If someone indicates ideation, respond with empathy, avoid judgment, and listen carefully. Also, try to make it easy for someone to respond affirmatively to your question. Saying "You're not suicidal, are you?" can shut the conversation off before it begins.

Supportive conversations can reduce the risk of suicide. The aim is not to diagnose, but to listen and maintain connection. According to the IPTS, feelings of thwarted belongingness and burdensomeness contribute to suicidal desire (Joiner, 2005; Van Orden et al. 2010). Calm, non-judgmental listening can reduce both. A supportive peer can foster a sense of connection and belonging while empathically challenging perceptions of being a burden. In Story 5.1, a veterinarian recounts how her mentor helped her during a crisis, even though they did not specifically discuss suicidality. The connection and the support were the most important factors in getting that veterinarian through that moment. This story also reflects the importance of means safety, which will be discussed in the next section.

Although suicide can follow a single difficult event, like the sudden loss of a loved one, it more often reflects a complex constellation of multiple stressors or long-standing problems (Fleischman et al. 2014). Exploring what has changed recently and what has "tipped the scales" helps guide support, but it may not explain the whole story. For example, in Story 5.2, a vet student experiences a minor setback that triggers severe ideation. However, in the background, multiple factors were at play. Without addressing these issues holistically, the underlying distress is likely to continue.

While discussing stressful circumstances and experiences, it can be helpful to ask about supportive relationships, previously effective coping strategies, and reasons for living (family, pets, etc.; CDC 2024). Encouraging individuals to identify their own coping strategies may also bolster

Table 5.2 Suicide Intervention_Asking the question

When asking if someone is experiencing suicidal thoughts, it's important to approach the conversation thoughtfully, with language that is supportive, rather than judgmental.
"Sometimes people who are feeling very overwhelmed and depressed have thoughts about suicide. Is that something you've been thinking about?"
"You have mentioned a few times how you can't go on. Sometimes people say that when they are having suicidal thoughts. Are you having suicidal thoughts?"
"I noticed that you said you don't want to live like this anymore. I completely understand feeling upset and overwhelmed with everything that's happening. I just wanted to clarify, does that mean you are having suicidal thoughts?"
"Hey, you've mentioned a lot of really hard situations. It seems like a lot to deal with, and I can understand feeling pretty overwhelmed. I just wanted to check in with you- are you having any suicidal thoughts?"

STORY 5.1 AN EQUINE VET REACHES OUT FOR SUPPORT

It was April of 2019, and I was in the final stretch of a year-long equine internship. Being an equine internist was all I had wanted for as long as I could remember, and I was absolutely devoted to it. My internship had been brutal. After 11 months of working more hours than anyone should physically work, enduring emotional abuse at the hands of my colleagues, packing trauma after trauma away, and being twisted and bent until I no longer recognized myself, I broke.

It was a warm morning, and I was standing outside the isolation stall in full gear. I needed to care for my patient, a young horse with raging colitis. He was so sick. And nothing I had done for him, day and night for almost 2 weeks, was helping. His head hung low. He burned with fever between each dose of NSAIDs. He smelled as though he had already died. In hindsight, he was symbolic of a war we were both losing.

I hadn't slept more than a few hours in the preceding three or four days. I don't remember much about what happened. I found myself sitting down on an overturned bucket, staring at my hands. I could not move. I was soaked with sweat and tears. Drowning in them.

I remember thinking: "He needs you. They need you. Just stand up." I wanted so badly to help him. But all I felt capable of was staring at my hands and picturing there, my pistol. And I hated myself for it. I honestly don't know that I would be here today if that gun hadn't been far from me in that moment.

In that moment, sitting on that bucket, I texted my mentor. She was caring and protective. I didn't tell her what was happening, but I think she inferred and helped talk me down. I'll always be grateful to her for that.

I passively considered killing myself, every day, for the next few months. It was comforting to contemplate an escape from what my life had become.

I had no prior history of mental health struggles or suicidal ideation. And none since. Now that I have some distance, I suppose the combination of sleep deprivation, chronic verbal abuse, and feelings of inadequacy could bring anyone to their knees.

STORY 5.2 A SMALL INCIDENT TRIGGERS IDEATION

I had struggled with depression, anxiety, and occasional ideation since I was a teenager. It was usually low-grade or not even there. Vet school really challenged my mental health, though. It brought out a pretty nasty, competitive, perfectionistic side of me that was not helping my depression and anxiety. Add to that, my husband, who had been my rock for seven years, moved to another country for work. I had a new roommate who I really wasn't getting along with, and money was tight. I was a fourth-year student in clinics, so I was generally overworked and exhausted. It was my clinical pathology rotation, probably one of the least stressful rotations. During it, we were supposed to do this small, casual presentation. It wasn't even graded. I bombed it. I got tongue-tied, couldn't remember anything, and generally freaked out. My ideation instantly got very loud. This presentation literally had no consequences, but screwing it up made me absolutely convinced I was a worthless failure. I couldn't think of anything else. I couldn't calm down. I was pretty sure that if I went home, I would hurt myself. So, instead, I walked into student health and asked to see someone. I'm super grateful to the counselor who fit me in that day. He probably saved my life.

feelings of autonomy, which has been associated with more effective intervention (Knapp et al. 2024). When people are involved in choosing coping strategies and supports that are meaningful to them, they are more likely to disclose distress and engage in help-seeking, which can reduce risk for suicide (Knapp et al. 2024). The simple question, "What have you tried so far?" can be a great conversation starter.

While a single conversation can be helpful, follow-up check-ins are also important. A meta-analysis found that regular follow-ups after crisis care reduced the number of repeated attempts (Inagaki et al. 2019). In personal settings, brief check-ins every few days are often feasible and help maintain connection during recovery. Remember that a person in crisis may not have the mental wherewithal to reach out to you or may mistakenly wish to avoid "burdening" their loved ones; don't just assume that everything is ok if you haven't received a direct request for help. By checking in, you are showing that you are not scared of having difficult conversations and that you are available for support over the long haul.

MEANS SAFETY

As we have discussed above, access to lethal means is a well-established risk factor for suicide, particularly in healthcare settings (Milner 2017). In veterinary medicine, self-poisoning is one of the most common methods of suicide (Tomasi, 2019). Pentobarbital is the most common substance used by veterinarians, whereas opioid poisoning is more frequently reported among technicians and technologists (Witte 2019; Tomasi 2019). Firearms are also a common method, with male veterinarians more likely to die by firearm (51%) than female veterinarians, who were more likely to die by self-poisoning (64%) (Tomasi 2019). This differs from the pattern seen in the general population, for whom firearms are the most common suicide method (53%), and self-poisoning is less common (9%; SPRC 2025). The overall pattern of findings is consistent with the notion that access to and knowledge about lethal drugs in the workplace may account, in part, for the elevated risk for suicide seen in veterinary professionals. Therefore, access to both lethal medications and firearms should be specifically addressed when assessing risk in veterinary professionals.

Means safety is an important part of suicide prevention. It involves restricting or delaying access to lethal methods, either temporarily or permanently. This strategy is sometimes met with resistance as people incorrectly believe that a suicidal person will simply find another method. To that point, in a focus group of veterinarians, concerns about practicality and effectiveness of means safety were common (Waitz-Kudla et al., 2023). However, means safety has consistently reduced suicide rates. For example, bans on lethal pesticides in several Asian countries resulted in a reduction of national suicide rates by 50% or more (Hawton et al. 2024). After firearm restrictions in Switzerland, only 22% of individuals sought alternative methods, and when they did, the chosen methods were less lethal (Reisch et al. 2013; Barber and Miller 2014).

In veterinary medicine, complete restriction is not always practical because access to two of the most common methods – firearms and controlled drugs – may be required for clinical work (Witte 2019). Thankfully, partial restriction can still have significant effects. Suicidal behavior is often impulsive, and suicidal crises tend to be short-lived. In several studies, about half of attempt survivors reported less than 10 minutes between the onset of suicidal intent and the attempt, and about one-third reported less than five minutes (Deisenhammer et al. 2009; Paashaus et al. 2021). A brief delay in access could therefore be life-saving.

Current storage practices suggest areas for improvement. Only 50% of veterinarian firearm owners in a focus group reported storing their firearms locked at all times, which presents an opportunity for an evidence-based, effective preventive measure (Waitz-Kudla et al., 2023; Roarke 2019). In this same study, 30% of veterinarians reported storing pentobarbital unlocked at least part of the time (Waitz-Kudla et a., 2023), and more than 70% of veterinary professionals reported they could access controlled drugs without another person present (Roarke 2019). How medications are stored also appears to influence suicidal planning. Individuals working in hospitals with unlocked access reported greater cognitive availability of lethal means, which mediated the relationship between recent ideation and perceived likelihood of future attempts (Houtsma et al. 2023). Practical storage strategies include two-person access systems (i.e. double lock boxes) and automated dispensing units (i.e. Cubex) that carefully track inventory and can require witness fingerprints to obtain medications. Organizational policies can also help create distance. For instance, a policy might require that the person ordering a medication is not the same as the person dispensing it, and that both parties be logged.

During periods of personal crisis, temporary adjustments can also be made. These may include decreasing contact with euthanasia solution by selective scheduling, or when euthanasia is unavoidable, by having a coworker draw up the drugs, bring them to the exam room, and witness the euthanasia. If firearms are required for ambulatory veterinarians, they can be stored locked away from the person in distress during non-work hours. While these adjustments do require planning and coordination, the benefits of safety are well worth that minor inconvenience.

SAFETY PLANNING

Planning around safety is not limited to restricting access to lethal means. Safety plans are written documents that outline what a person can do when suicidal thoughts increase. A typical safety plan lists warning signs, coping strategies for managing distress, supportive contacts to reach out to, and steps to reduce access to highly lethal methods. Plans are most effective when completed during periods of relative stability, written down, and shared with trusted supporters (Stanley and Brown 2012). Free templates are available at https://suicidesafetyplan.com and through the Suicide Safety Plan App.

Safety plans are understood to work through several mechanisms. In moments of crisis, suicidal thinking often becomes narrow and problem-solving ability decreases (Wenzel et al. 2009). A written sequence of steps provides structure and guidance when a person may be overwhelmed or unable to think clearly (Stanley and Brown 2012). Listing reasons for living, future goals, and supportive contacts helps counter hopelessness and isolation, which are known drivers of suicidal desire (Van Orden 2010).

There is growing evidence that safety plans are effective. A meta-analysis found that safety plan interventions reduced suicidal behavior by approximately 43% and also improved depression and hopelessness (Nuij et al. 2021). These reductions occurred even when individuals continued to experience suicidal ideation, indicating that the presence of suicidal thoughts does not make safety planning futile. Safety plans, therefore, represent a brief, practical, and evidence-based tool that can be used in clinical settings, workplaces, and personal support networks.

EMERGENCY SERVICES

Emergency services are important for individuals at imminent risk, such as those with suicidal intent, detailed plans, access to lethal means, or no ability to remain safe. However, most crises do not require involuntary intervention. Data from the National Suicide Prevention Lifeline show that fewer than 1% of calls lead to emergency services being contacted without the callers' consent and cooperation (Wortzel et al., 2019). If emergency services are necessary, involve the person in decision-making, maintain autonomy, and use the least intrusive option that ensures safety. In some areas, mobile crisis teams or psychiatric emergency units can respond to mental health crises (NRI 2023). Along those lines, approximately one-third of mental health treatment facilities offer walk-in emergency services (SAMHSA 2021; Rodriguez 2023), and a growing number of areas have access to mental health urgent-care clinics (AAMC 2024). These providers offer more assured access to trained mental health professionals than standard emergency rooms (AAMC 2024). Of course, it is important to be aware that the availability of these services varies by region and may not be an option in your area.

Hospitalization may become necessary for high-risk individuals, particularly when there is immediate danger. However, involuntary admission can be distressing, and studies have reported iatrogenic effects such as fear, reduced trust, and avoidance of future care (Ward-Ciesielski and Rizvi 2021). There is also an elevated risk of suicide in the weeks following psychiatric discharge (Hunt et al., 2009, Hjorthøj et al., 2014). However, it is unclear whether this reflects the effects of hospitalization or the severity of underlying illness. When hospital care is needed, explaining what will happen, remaining with the person if possible, helping them contact trusted supports, and ensuring continuity of care can reduce distress and improve outcomes.

WHEN YOU ARE THE ONE AT RISK

Veterinary professionals are often highly empathic, and it is common to put the needs of others first, even when their own well-being is suffering (Laura et al. 2024). Much of this chapter has focused on how to recognize and respond to suicidal risk in others, but that same care applies to ourselves. Airline safety instructions remind us, "put your own oxygen mask on first" because you cannot safely care for others if you are in danger yourself.

Suicidal thoughts are not a sign of weakness or failure; they are a signal of distress that can improve with support. If these thoughts appear, reaching out to a trusted person, a mental health professional, or a crisis service is an important step in staying safe. The strategies described in this chapter, such as reducing access to lethal means, creating a safety plan, and seeking connection, can be used for self-care as well as for helping others. Research consistently shows that even a brief human connection can reduce suicidal intensity and improve coping (Inagaki et al. 2019; Nuij et al. 2021). Veterinary-specific support services are listed in Table 5.3. Please note that most of these are not crisis lines with help available 24/7 but can provide veterinary-specific resources. Many of these organizations also provided continuing education content, which can be found on their websites. If you or someone else is in need of urgent help, Table 5.4 has a list of crisis services available in the United States. For readers outside the United States, Befrienders Worldwide maintains an international directory of crisis and emotional support services (www.befrienders.org).

Table 5.3 Veterinary-specific support resources

Resource	Who it serves	How to access	Availability / format
Vetlife Helpline (UK)	Veterinary professionals in the UK and Ireland	https://helpline.vetlife.org.uk	Phone support 24/7; email replies typically within 24 hours
Veterinary Hope	Veterinary professionals in various areas of practice	https://www.veterinaryhope.org/community-groups	Mental health professional–led groups with scheduled start dates
NOMV Lifeboat	Veterinary professionals	https://nomv.org/peer-support/#Lifeboat	Anonymous peer support; typically matched within ~48 hours
NOMV Veterinary Mental Health Support (VMHS)	Veterinary professionals in various areas of practice	Email VMHS@nomv.org	Scheduled groups, individual sessions, and monthly webinars
AVA Telephone Counselling Service (Thrive)	AVA members, staff, and family members (Australia)	Call 1300 687 327	24/7 confidential service providing individualized referrals and practical action plans
VIN Foundation Vets4Vets and Support4Support	Veterinarians and veterinary support staff	https://vinfoundation.org/resources/vets4vets/	One-on-one peer support matched to individual needs

Table 5.4 Crisis resources in the United States

Resource	Who it serves	How to access	Availability	Notes
988 Suicide and Crisis Lifeline	Anyone in the United States	Call or text 988	24/7	National network of crisis lines
Crisis Text Line	Anyone in the United States	Text HOME to 741741	24/7	Crisis line staffed by trained volunteers
BlackLine	Black, Indigenous, and People of Color (BIPOC) callers	Call or text 1-844-460-7225	24/7	Culturally responsive crisis and peer support
Trans Lifeline	Transgender and questioning individuals	Call 877-565-8860	Open Mon-Fri 10 AM –6 PM Pacific	Peer support staffed by trans operators
LGBT National Help Center	LGBTQ people of all ages	Call 1-888-843-4564	Open Mon-Fri 11 AM–8 PM, Sat 9am–2pm Pacific time	Confidential peer support, information, and referrals

For readers outside the United States, Befrienders Worldwide maintains an international directory of crisis and emotional support services (www.befrienders.org).

CONCLUSION

Suicide prevention in veterinary medicine begins with acknowledging the reality of elevated risk and the unique occupational pressures that contribute to it. Factors like exposure to euthanasia can increase vulnerability, yet none of these factors make suicide inevitable. Indeed, it is important to keep in mind that suicide remains mercifully rare in veterinary professionals – having approximately double the risk of a very rare outcome in the general population is something that warrants appropriate attention and concern, but not panic.

That perspective exists alongside another reality. Veterinary medicine is a relatively small field. While there are just under one million physicians and over four million registered nurses in the United States, there are just over 130,000 veterinarians and a similar number of veterinary technicians (AVMA 2024; BLS 2024; NCSBN 2024). In a profession of this size, news of a death by suicide can be far-reaching, quickly moving through overlapping professional and social networks and raising awareness of the tragedy. In an informal poll conducted within the Not One More Vet online support group (n = 1,218), 71% of veterinarian respondents reported personally knowing someone in the field who had died by suicide (NOMV 2025). Although this informal poll is not peer reviewed and likely reflects the self-selected nature of a support-focused community, it nonetheless illustrates how closely suicide touches many veterinary professionals, even as the events themselves remain statistically rare.

Connection, support, treatment, and practical strategies matter. Evidence-based approaches such as means safety, safety planning, empathetic communication, and regular follow-up help reduce both intent and opportunity for harm, even when suicidal thoughts persist. At its core, prevention is about staying present. A single compassionate conversation can interrupt a crisis, and a brief moment of human connection can help someone feel less alone. Whether we are responding to a colleague, a friend, or ourselves, we do not need to solve everything at once. We only need to create safety long enough for hope, help, and healing to remain possible.

REFERENCES

American Veterinary Medical Association (AVMA). (2024). *Market research statistics: U.S. veterinarians.* https://www.avma.org/resources-tools/reports-statistics/market-research-statistics-us-veterinarians/ (accessed 12 January 2026).

Andreo-Jover, J., Ramos, J.C., Bobes, J. et al. (2024). The mediating role of reflective functioning in the association between childhood trauma and suicide attempt. *Journal of Psychiatric Research* 171: 30–37.

Association of American Medical Colleges (AAMC) (2024) 'Walk-in clinics tackle urgent mental health needs'. https://www.aamc.org/news/walk-clinics-tackle-urgent-mental-health-needs (accessed 9 January 2026).

Baca-García, E., Perez-Rodriguez, M.M., Oquendo, M.A. et al. (2008). Estimating risk for suicide attempt: are we asking the right questions? *Journal of Affective Disorders* 107 (1-3): 107–114.

Bader, S., Abbes, W., Tfifha, M., et al. 2021. Warning signs of suicide attempts and risk of suicidal recurrence. *European Psychiatry*, 64, pp. S589–S589. https://doi.org/10.1192/j.eurpsy.2021.1571.

Barber, C.W. and Miller, M.J. (2014). Reducing a suicidal person's access to lethal means of suicide: a research agenda. *American Journal of Preventive Medicine* 47 (3): S264–S272.

Bartram, D.J. and Baldwin, D.S. (2010). Veterinary surgeons and suicide: a structured review of possible influences on increased risk. *Veterinary Record* 166 (13): 388–397.

Blair, A. and Hayes, H.M. Jr. (1982). Mortality patterns among U.S. veterinarians, 1947–1977: an expanded study. *International Journal of Epidemiology* 11 (4): 391–397.

Bostwick, J.M., Pabbati, C., Geske, J.R., and McKean, A.J. (2016). Suicide attempt as a risk factor for completed suicide: even more lethal than we knew. *American Journal of Psychiatry* 173 (11): 1094–1100.

Bryan, C.J., Allen, M.H., Wastler, H.M. et al. (2023). Rapid intensification of suicide risk preceding suicidal behavior among primary care patients. *Suicide and Life-Threatening Behavior* 53 (3): 352–361.

Bureau of Labor Statistics, U.S. Department of Labor (BLS), 2024. Occupational outlook handbook, veterinary technologists and technicians. https://www.bls.gov/ooh/healthcare/veterinary-technologists-and-technicians.htm (accessed 12 November 2025).

Cai, Z., Junus, A., Chang, Q., and Yip, P.S. (2022). The lethality of suicide methods: a systematic review and meta-analysis. *Journal of Affective Disorders* 300: 121–129.

CDC, 2022. Suicide data and statistics. Centers for Disease Control and Prevention. https://www.cdc.gov/ (accessed 27 December 2024).

Centers for Disease Control and Prevention (2024) Risk and protective factors for suicide [Online]. https://www.cdc.gov/suicide/risk-factors/index.html (accessed 12 November 2025).

Chan, C.K. and Wong, P.W. (2023). Predictors of suicide risk and mental health outcomes among Hong Kong veterinarians: a cross-sectional study. *Behavioral Sciences* 13 (9): 770.

Chu, C., Klein, K.M., Buchman-Schmitt, J.M. et al. (2015). Routinized assessment of suicide risk in clinical practice: an empirically informed update. *Journal of Clinical Psychology* 71 (12): 1186–1200.

da Silva, C.R., Gomes, A.A.D., dos Santos-Doni, T.R. et al. (2023). Suicide in veterinary medicine: a literature review. *Veterinary World* 16 (6): 1266.

Dalum, H.S., Tyssen, R., Moum, T. et al. (2024). Euthanasia of animals and veterinarians' suicidal thoughts: a nationwide cross-sectional study (the NORVET study). *BMC Psychiatry* 24 (1): 2.

Daray, F.M., Grendas, L.N., Neupane, S.P. et al. (2025). Prediction of fatal and non-fatal suicide attempts by the Columbia Suicide Severity Rating Scale (C-SSRS): systematic review and meta-analysis. *The British Journal of Psychiatry* 1–14.

Deisenhammer, E.A., Ing, C.-M., Strauss, R. et al. (2009). The duration of the suicidal process: how much time is left for intervention between consideration and accomplishment of a suicide attempt? *Journal of Clinical Psychiatry* 70 (1): 19–24.

Ferm, M.S., Frazee, L.A., Kennard, B.D. et al. (2020). Fearlessness about death predicts adolescent suicide attempt: a preliminary analysis. *Suicide and Life-Threatening Behavior* 50 (6): 1288–1295.

Fleischmann, A., Howlader, S., Vijayakumar, L., and Butchart, A. (2014). *Preventing Suicide: A Global Imperative*. Luxembourg: World Health Organization.

Have, M.T., De Graaf, R., Van Dorsselaer, S. et al. (2009). Incidence and course of suicidal ideation and suicide attempts in the general population. *The Canadian Journal of Psychiatry* 54 (12): 824–833.

Hawton, K., Bergen, H., Simkin, S. et al. (2013). Effect of pesticide regulation on suicide in Sri Lanka. *BJPsych* 203 (5): 386–392.

Hawton, K., Knipe, D., and Pirkis, J. (2024). Restriction of access to means used for suicide. *The Lancet Public Health* 9 (10): e796–e801.

Hill, E.M., LaLonde, C., and Wilson, J. (2020). Euthanasia-related strain among veterinary technicians. *Frontiers in Veterinary Science* 7: 578.

Hjorthøj, C.R., Madsen, T., Agerbo, E., and Nordentoft, M. (2014). Risk of suicide according to level of psychiatric treatment: a nationwide nested case–control study. *Social Psychiatry and Psychiatric Epidemiology* 49 (9): 1357–1365.

Houtsma, C., Bond, A.E., and Anestis, M.D. (2023). Access to lethal means and suicidal planning among healthcare workers. *Psychiatry Research* 27 (4): 1351–1362.

Hunt, I.M., Kapur, N., Webb, R. et al. (2009). Suicide in recently discharged psychiatric patients: a case-control study. *Psychological Medicine* 39 (3): 443–449.

Inagaki, M., Kawashima, Y., Yonemoto, N., and Yamada, M. (2019). Active contact and follow-up interventions to prevent repeat suicide attempts during high-risk periods among patients admitted to emergency departments for suicidal behavior: a systematic review and meta-analysis. *BMC Psychiatry* 19 (1): 44.

Joiner, T.E. (2005). *Why People Die by Suicide*. Cambridge, MA: Harvard University Press.

Kinlen, L.J. (1983). Mortality among British veterinary surgeons. *British Medical Journal* 287 (6398): 1017.

Klonsky, E.D. and May, A.M. (2015). The Three-Step Theory (3ST): a new theory of suicide. *Clinical Psychological Science* 3 (2): 189–203.

Klonsky, E.D., May, A.M., and Saffer, B.Y. (2014). Suicide, suicide attempts, and suicidal ideation. *Annual Review of Clinical Psychology* 10: 307–330.

Knapp, S.J. (2024). Listen, explain, involve, and evaluate: Why respecting autonomy benefits suicidal patients. *Ethics & Behavior* 34 (1): 18–27.

Kogan, L.R., Wallace, J.E., Schoenfeld-Tacher, R. et al. (2020). Veterinary technicians and occupational burnout. *Frontiers in Veterinary Science* 7: 328.

Laura, L., Arapović, M., Duvnjak, S., and Arapović, J. (2024). Empathy and mental health in veterinary medicine. *Veterinary Research Communications* 48 (4): 1991–1997.

Lerner, H., Lindblad, A., Algers, B., and Lynöe, N. (2011). Veterinary surgeons' attitudes towards physician-assisted suicide: an empirical study of Swedish experts on euthanasia. *Journal of Medical Ethics* 37 (5): 295–298.

Milner, A., Witt, K., Maheen, H., and LaMontagne, A.D. (2017). Access to means of suicide and occupation: a national study over 12 years of coronial data. *BMC Psychiatry* 17: 1–7.

Milner, A., Witt, K., Maheen, H., and LaMontagne, A.D. (2017). Access to means of suicide, occupation and the risk of suicide: a national study over 12 years of coronial data. *BMC psychiatry* 17 (1): 125.

Moses, L., Malowney, M., and Wesley Boyd, J. (2018). Ethical conflict and euthanasia in veterinary medicine. *Journal of the American Veterinary Medical Association* 252 (2): 151–158.

National Council of State Boards of Nursing (NCSBN) (2024). *2024 NCSBN Workforce Survey: Infographic*. Chicago, IL: NCSBN. https://www.ncsbn.org/public-files/2024-NCSBN-WorkforceSurvey-Infographic.pdf.

National Research Institute, Inc. (NRI) (2023). *Profiles: mobile crisis teams 2023*. https://nri-inc.org/media/m4sgp1mp/profiles-mobile-crisis-teams-2023.pdf.

Nett, R.J., Witte, T.K., Holzbauer, S.M. et al. (2015). Risk factors for suicide, attitudes toward mental illness, and practice-related stressors among US veterinarians. *Journal of the American Veterinary Medical Association* 247 (8): 945–955.

Nett, R.J., Witte, T.K., Holzbauer, S.M. et al. (2015). Risk factors for suicide, attitudes toward mental illness, and practice-related stressors among US veterinarians. *Journal of the American Veterinary Medical Association* 247 (8): 945–955.

Nett, R.J., Witte, T.K., Tomasi, S.E., and Fowler, K.A. (2020). Storage of euthanasia solution as a factor in addressing veterinarian suicides. *Journal of the American Veterinary Medical Association* 256 (12): 1321–1322.

Nett, R.J., Witte, T.K., Tomasi, S.E., and Fowler, K.A. (2020). Storage of euthanasia solution as a factor in addressing veterinarian suicides. *Journal of the American Veterinary Medical Association* 256 (12): 1321–1322.

Nock, M.K., Borges, G., Bromet, E.J. et al. (2008). Suicide and suicidal behavior. *Epidemiologic Reviews* 30 (1): 133–154.

Not One More Vet (NOMV) (2025). Facebook poll post: "How many of you know someone personally from our field who has died by suicide?" [Online poll]. Facebook, 12 October 2025. https://www.facebook.com/groups/NOMVet/posts/4212223668991251 (accessed 12 January 2026).

Nuij, C., Van Ballegooijen, W., De Beurs, D. et al. (2021). Safety planning-type interventions for suicide prevention: meta-analysis. *The British Journal of Psychiatry* 219 (2): 419–426.

O'Connor, R.C. (2011). The integrated motivational–volitional model of suicidal behaviour. *Crisis* 32 (6): 295–298.

Olfson, M., Cosgrove, C.M., Wall, M.M., and Blanco, C. (2023). Suicide risks of health care workers in the US. *JAMA* 330 (12): 1161–1166.

Owens, D., Horrocks, J., and House, A. (2002). Fatal and non-fatal repetition of self-harm. *British Journal of Psychiatry* 181: 193–199.

Paashaus, L., Forkmann, T., Glaesmer, H. et al. (2021). Suicidal impulse and rapid onset of attempts. *Journal of Affective Disorders* 286: 77–84.

Platt, B., Hawton, K., Simkin, S. et al. (2012). Suicidality in the veterinary profession. In: *Crisis*.

Pompili, M., Murri, M.B., Patti, S. et al. (2016). Communication of suicidal intent: a systematic review. *Crisis* 37 (5): 359–368.

Posner, K., Brown, G.K., Stanley, B. et al. (2011). The Columbia–Suicide Severity Rating Scale: initial validity and internal consistency findings from three multisite studies with adolescents and adults. *American Journal of Psychiatry* 168 (12): 1266–1277.

Prabhakar, D., Peterson, E.L., Hu, Y. et al. (2020). Serious suicide attempts and risk of suicide death. *Crisis* 42 (5): 343–350.

Reisch, T., Steffen, T., Habenstein, A., and Tschacher, W. (2013). Decrease in suicide by firearms after firearm restriction in Switzerland. *American Journal of Psychiatry* 170 (9): 977–984.

Roarke, A., 2019. What do we do about suicide? it's time to limit access to means. https://drandyroark.com/what-do-we-do-about-suicide/ (accessed 27 December 2024).

Rodriguez, T. (2023). Current state of emergency mental health care in the US. *Psychiatry Advisor.* https://www.psychiatryadvisor.com/features/many-areas-in-us-lack-access-to-emergency-psychiatric-and-crisis-services/ (accessed 9 January 2026).

Rudd, M.D., Berman, A.L., Joiner, T.E. Jr. et al. (2006). Warning signs for suicide: theory, research, and clinical applications. *Suicide and Life-Threatening Behavior* 36 (3): 255–262.

Salway, T., Ross, L.E., Fehr, C.P. et al. (2019). Disparities in suicide ideation and attempt among bisexual populations. *Archives of Sexual Behavior* 48: 89–111.

Schunter, N., Glaesmer, H., Lucht, L., and Bahramsoltani, M. (2022). Depression, suicidal ideation and suicide risk in German veterinary medical students compared to the German general population. *PLOS One* 17 (8): e0270912.

Scoresby, K., Jurney, C., Fackler, A. et al. (2023). Diversity demographics, psychological distress, and suicidal thinking in the veterinary profession. *Frontiers in Veterinary Science* 10: 1130826.

Shanafelt, T.D., Balch, C.M., Dyrbye, L. et al. (2011). Suicidal ideation among American surgeons. *Archives of Surgery* 146 (1): 54–62.

Stanley, B. and Brown, G. (2012). Safety planning intervention: a brief intervention to mitigate suicide risk. *Cognitive and Behavioral Practice* 19 (2): 256–264.

Substance Abuse and Mental Health Services Administration (SAMHSA) (2021). *National Mental Health Services Survey (N-MHSS): 2020. Data on Mental Health Treatment Facilities*. Rockville, MD: SAMHSA. https://www.samhsa.gov/data/sites/default/files/reports/rpt35336/2020_NMHSS_final.pdf.

Suicide Prevention Resource Center (SPRC) (2025) Means of suicide: scope of the problem. https://sprc.org/about-suicide/scope-of-the-problem/means-of-suicide/ (accessed 9 January 2026).

Teismann, T., Siebert, A.M., and Forkmann, T. (2024). Suicidal ambivalence: a scoping review. *Suicide and Life-Threatening Behavior* 54 (5): 802–813.

Tomasi, S.E., Fechter-Leggett, E.D., Edwards, N.T. et al. (2019). Suicide among veterinarians in the United States from 1979 through 2015. *Journal of the American Veterinary Medical Association* 254 (1): 104–112.

Tomasi, S.E., Fechter-Leggett, E.D., Edwards, N.T. et al. (2019). Suicide among veterinarians in the United States from 1979 through 2015. *Journal of the American Veterinary Medical Association* 254 (1): 104–112.

Van Orden, K.A., Witte, T.K., Cukrowicz, K.C. et al. (2010). The interpersonal theory of suicide. *Psychological Review* 117 (2): 575–600.

Waitz-Kudla, S.N., Kramper, S., Roark, A. et al. (2023). Securing lethal means for suicide: a focus group study among practicing veterinarians. *Journal of the American Veterinary Medical Association* 261 (11): 1683–1693.

Wall, M., Schenck-Gustafsson, K., Minucci, D. et al. (2014). Suicidal ideation among surgeons in Italy and Sweden. *BMC Psychology* 2: 1–8.

Ward-Ciesielski, E.F. and Rizvi, S.L. (2021). The potential iatrogenic effects of psychiatric hospitalization for suicidal behavior: a critical review and recommendations for research. *Clinical Psychology: Science and Practice* 28 (1): 60.

Wenzel, A., Brown, G.K., and Beck, A.T. (2009). *Cognitive Therapy for Suicidal Patients: Scientific and Clinical Applications*. Washington, DC: American Psychological Association.

Witte, T.K., Correia, C.J., and Angarano, D. (2013). Experience with euthanasia is associated with fearlessness about death in veterinary students. *Suicide and Life-Threatening Behavior* 43 (2): 125–138.

Witte, T.K., Spitzer, E.G., Edwards, N. et al. (2019). Suicides and deaths of undetermined intent among veterinary professionals from 2003 through 2014. *Journal of the American Veterinary Medical Association* 255 (5): 595–608.

World Health Organization (WHO), 2014. Preventing suicide: A global imperative. World Health Organization. https://www.who.int/publications/i/item/9789241564779 (accessed 9 January 2025)

Wortzel, H.S., Barnes, S.M., Cannizzaro, K.A., et al. (2019) Welfare checks and therapeutic risk management. Journal of Psychiatric Practice, 25(6), pp. 470–474. https://doi.org/10.1097/PRA.0000000000000434

Waitz-Kudla, S.N., Kramper, S., Roark, A. et al. (2023). Securing lethal means for suicide: a focus group study exploring perceptions and barriers among practicing veterinarians. *Journal of the American Veterinary Medical Association* 261 (11): 1683–1693.

Van Orden, K.A., Witte, T.K., Cukrowicz, K.C. et al. (2010). The interpersonal theory of suicide. *Psychological review* 117 (2): 575.

Yip, P.S.F., Gunnell, D., Fang, Y.Y. et al. (2012). Means restriction for suicide prevention and implications. *The Lancet* 379 (9834): 2395–2405.

Zakharankov, A. (2023). The emotional toll of financial stress, work environment, and euthanasia: third annual veterinary burnout survey. *Galaxy Vets.* https://links.galaxyvets.com/burnoutstudy (accessed 27 December 2024).

Professional Stressors

CHAPTER 6

Carrie Jurney, DVM, DACVIM (Neurology)[1] and Sharon Kramper, PhD[2]

[1] *Not One More Vet, Inc, San Francisco, CA, USA*
[2] *Northwestern University Feinberg School of Medicine, Chicago, IL, USA*

INTRODUCTION

More than 80% of veterinarians agree that veterinary medicine is stressful. However, 80% of that same group of veterinarians also said that they enjoy their work (Robinson et al. 2019). On the surface, these two statements appear contradictory. Instead, it demonstrates the complexity of happiness. As discussed in Chapter 1, happiness is not simply the lack of stress, nor is it solely dependent on indulgent pleasures. Prominent researchers and philosophers share the view that true happiness includes the satisfaction of meaningful work. The pursuit of meaningful work is not always pleasant and can certainly be fraught with long hours and a variety of other unpleasant things. That being said, meaningful work has also been found to be one of the strongest predictors of veterinary well-being (Cake et al. 2015; Wallace 2019). To connect with the fulfillment and satisfaction that come with meaningful work, we need to learn to mitigate the negative aspects as much as possible.

Several researchers in veterinary well-being have cautioned against a negative focus. They suggest that this draws our focus to just the downsides of the profession (Cake et al. 2015; Wallace 2019). Given the profession's tendency towards neuroticism, you can understand why focusing on negative aspects of well-being might be tempting and, indeed, could create a self-fulfilling prophecy. However, just as we cannot discuss treatment without discussing pathophysiology, we can't consider well-being without considering where it can go off the rails. Successfully navigating a veterinary career requires recognizing the stressors we commonly face and the coping skills needed to manage them.

Many stressors in veterinary medicine cannot be fully removed. For instance, no matter how many stress-free handling classes we take, at some point, an animal will lash out in fear, and you might get injured. That does not mean we should not work towards safer animal handling. We cannot let perfectionism constrain us to unrealistic goals. Instead, we must be mindful of our challenges and the impacts they have on us, while working on mitigation strategies that may be imperfect. In this chapter, we will review the most common professional stressors and strategies to help veterinary professionals cope with them. We will discuss stressors inherent to the work of veterinary professionals that are largely independent of our particular workplace. Stressors that are tied to the culture and structure of your specific practice, such as work hours, will be covered in Chapter 7.

INTERPERSONAL RELATIONSHIPS AND CONFLICT

Veterinary professionals often say they like animals more than people. However, animal patients are not capable of making, attending, nor paying for their appointments unsupervised, so some human contact is required. Aside from client interactions, we also interact daily with management, coworkers, and colleagues, and each interaction presents an opportunity for conflict. In a survey of UK veterinarians, a majority of respondents reported that working with pet owners was stressful, and one-third reported that their interpersonal relationships with colleagues were also stressful (O'Connor 2019). In a survey of veterinarians in the United States, respondents cited client complaints as one of the reasons they considered leaving the profession, demonstrating that interpersonal relationships are a prominent stressor in the veterinary field (Nett et al. 2015).

CONFLICT WITH CLIENTS

Conflict with clients can take many forms, ranging from brief, unpleasant interactions to formal complaints, lawsuits, and even threats of physical harm. In surveys of veterinary professionals, a majority of veterinarians and one-third of veterinary support staff reported receiving a client complaint regarding their work in the last six months (Bryce 2019; Rogers et al. 2022). Approximately one-third of complaints directed at veterinarians involved verbal abuse and/or threats of litigation (Bryce 2019). The consequences reported by the recipients of these complaints included depression, negative impacts on job enjoyment, and alterations in medical practice made purely to avoid conflict. Most concerningly, a significant number of individuals – 43.5% of veterinarians and 26.5% of staff – considered a career change after these complaints (Bryce 2019).

A review of professional negligence claims to a veterinary liability insurance provider indicated that 80% of client conflict cases involve a communication breakdown, either between the owner and practitioner directly (49.4%) or between veterinary team members (42.3%; Russell et al. 2022). For instance, an owner may not feel they understood the potential complications of a surgery and feel deceived when a complication occurs. These findings suggest a point of intervention. Improved communication pathways, be they rounds among clinical staff or detailed forms discussing surgical complications, are a pathway to improved communication and decreased conflict.

CONFLICT WITH COWORKERS AND MANAGEMENT

Coworkers can also be a source of conflict, which may escalate if left unaddressed. In a survey of veterinarians and RVTs, conflict avoidance was cited as a component of a "toxic attitude" in the workplace (Moore et al. 2015). The results also indicated that the presence of toxic personalities can lead to decreased work satisfaction and burnout, so it is important to address coworker conflict immediately and effectively.

In an ideal situation, senior colleagues or leadership would address conflicts. Unfortunately, leaders can be the source of the conflict. Moreover, conflict with a senior colleague has a significantly greater impact on well-being compared to conflict with a coworker. In a survey of 252 veterinary staff members in the United Kingdom, conflict with a senior colleague had approximately four times the impact on mental health, nine times the impact on job satisfaction, four times the impact on turnover intention, and more than double the impact on burnout (Irwin et al. 2022).

ADDRESSING CONFLICT

Because the veterinary profession involves frequent contact with others, the solution is to learn how to resolve conflicts effectively, whether with clients or coworkers. Adept conflict resolution differentiates a healthy workplace from a toxic one. By nature, conflicts are emotional, and emotional reactions do not always lead to the best solutions. Mindfulness and emotion regulation skills (discussed in Chapter 10) provide us with a skillset to recognize and examine our own feelings, rather than acting when we are emotionally overwhelmed.

Kwame Christian (2020), lawyer and director of the American Negotiation Institute, outlines a three-part strategy for addressing conflict: acknowledge emotions, engage in compassionate curiosity, and work to solve problems jointly. This might start with an empathetic statement, such as, "It seems like you might have been frustrated yesterday." This statement opens the door for the other party to explore their own emotions. Once emotions are addressed, introduce questions to understand the perspectives of all parties. These questions should be based in good intent, without making assumptions about the motivations of others. This process leads to a more complete understanding of the objective facts and perspectives that led to the conflict. Finally, once all that information has been collected, the parties work together to develop a solution.

CYBERBULLYING

The Internet provides a forum for clients to vent through online reviews and social media. A negative review, while unpleasant, can contain constructive and important feedback. The vast majority of veterinarians said that they both appreciate (97%) and act on (95%) feedback from clients that is provided constructively and respectfully (Pikel 2022). Even when reviews are not respectful, they rarely rise to the level of cyberbullying. The average negative review should be viewed and addressed like any other conflict: with empathy, curiosity, and communication. However, the person being reviewed is not necessarily the best person to navigate this emotional landscape. It can be helpful to have a trusted colleague, such as a practice manager, read these reviews, provide a summary, and discuss any actionable feedback. This person can also, if deemed necessary or appropriate, reach out to de-escalate the situation with the client. However, when negative interactions escalate beyond a single negative review, a different strategy is warranted.

Cyberbullying entails "willful and repeated harm" (Hinduja and Patchin 2014). A cyberbullying attack rises from a mere disagreement between a veterinary professional and a client to a coordinated attack with the intent to not only express displeasure but also to cause emotional, financial, and sometimes physical harm. Unfortunately, cyberbullying has increased over the last decade. In 2014, 20.8% of companion animal veterinarians polled by the AVMA had been either the primary victim of cyberbullying or knew of a colleague who experienced it. In 2022, that number rose to 40.6% (AVMA Cyberbullying 2022). Cyberbullying attacks include recruiting others to participate by posting repeated negative reviews on a business (i.e. "review bombing") or asking people to share a negative social media post. Unfortunately, anger tends to drive engagement, so negative content spreads faster and farther than positive, uplifting content. When negative content goes viral, the impact can be widespread (Chuai and Zhao 2022; Fan et al. 2018).

Cyberbullying is a concern even for those who are not personally the focus of an attack. Although only 20% of veterinarians polled in the Merck Wellbeing Study reported experiencing an attack in the last year, 70% consider it a critical issue facing our field (Volk et al. 2022). Witnessing a cyberbullying incident online can cause anger in defense of colleagues, even when we are not directly impacted. Thus, two strategies are needed as part of a professional skillset: one for witnesses and one for when we are personally attacked.

When we see content about our colleagues, the most important thing is not to engage on social media. It is a natural, even noble, impulse to defend a colleague. You may feel defensive not only on behalf of your colleague but also on behalf of the entire profession, including yourself. However, every comment, mention, and share of a post online only serves to boost the prominence of the original content. Instead, provide support in other forms, such as direct messages, positive reviews, and supportive comments in places other than the original attack. These actions can help balance the negative onslaught this person or clinic is experiencing.

When we are personally affected, it's very easy to feel overwhelmed, and the urge to defend ourselves might be high. However, an emotional response can fan the flames of the situation. The first step if you are the subject of an attack is to appoint another person who will respond strategically and unemotionally to lead the response. The point person will manage social media accounts and take relevant screenshots as documentation until the storm passes, while the target of the attack limits their contact with social media. All threats of violence should be reported to the authorities immediately. Report the attack to relevant social media and review sites, as coordinated attacks often violate their terms of service and may result in content removal. Ensure that staff monitoring emails or answering phones are aware of the situation and are prepared to answer questions in a calm and professional way. If a practice feels compelled to respond, especially if there is media coverage involved, it is highly recommended that they contact a Professional Relations (PR) professional or other cyberbullying resources before doing so. Resources can be found at https://www.nomv.org/anti-cyber-harassment/ or through other organizations such as the AVMA.

The majority of veterinarians (52.9%) experiencing cyberbullying attacks reported moderate to severe emotional distress, with one-third reporting some level of stress-induced physical harm, such as unintended weight loss or loss of sleep (AVMA Cyberbullying 2022). Team members can be affected, too; 24% of practices that have experienced cyberbullying lost staff as a result. Practices can mitigate this loss by clearly communicating the clinic's strategy and conveying support during these incidents to all team members (Pikel 2021, 2022). However, the majority of attacks have little to no impact on revenue (76.1%), and the effect is temporary for the vast majority of cases (AVMA 2021). Similarly, despite threats of reporting to licensing boards being a common component of these attacks, only a small minority (9.9%) actually proceed with formal board complaints (AVMA Cyberbullying 2022).

PROFESSIONAL STRESSORS

While a career in medicine offers fantastic opportunities to live a life of purpose and meaning, it also exposes practitioners to highly stressful events, including those classified as traumatic. Traumatic events are those that haunt practitioners afterward and involve experiencing serious injury or violence or being threatened with serious injury, violence, or death. At work, this could include being mauled by a dog, kicked by a horse, or witnessing a similar event happen to someone. In addition, exposure to gruesome cases can be considered traumatic. Due to the nature of the field, full avoidance of highly stressful circumstances is likely impossible, but the probability of these events and their impact can be mitigated.

RISKS TO PHYSICAL HEALTH AND SAFETY

Veterinary medicine is consistently ranked among the top five most dangerous professions for nonfatal illness and injury by the Occupational Safety and Health Administration (OSHA 2022). When asked, most veterinary professionals can readily point to scars on their bodies or tell harrowing stories of times when they just barely got away. Health and safety hazards are numerous and include repetitive strain injury, needlesticks, animal bites, cuts from a scalpel blade, and zoonotic diseases.

In a survey of Utah veterinarians, 60% reported a needlestick, 40% an animal bite, 20% had been cut with a scalpel blade or necropsy knife, 22% had contracted a zoonotic disease, and 67% of those who frequently palpated large animals experienced joint pain (Rood and Pate 2019). Underlying these rather alarming injury rates, hand hygiene and sharps management were shown to be inconsistent at best. Only 51% reported washing their hands consistently before eating or drinking, and even fewer (35.6%) did so between patients; 67% reported recapping needles; and 55% reported eating and drinking in animal handling areas. General Personal Protective Equipment (PPE) use (gloves, face shields, etc.) was low, except during surgical procedures (Rood and Pate 2019). It would appear that a cultural shift within veterinary medicine is needed with an eye toward preventative measures.

While accidents will happen, we are not powerless to prevent them. Improvements have been validated in human medicine, and veterinary medicine would likely benefit from adopting them. Historically, hand hygiene compliance in human medicine was similar to that reported in veterinary medicine at 40% (Lotfinejad et al. 2021). However, with the implementation of hand hygiene programs, such as the WHO Five Moments for Hand Hygiene campaign (https://www.who.int/publications/m/item/five-moments-for-hand-hygiene) and the use of alcohol-based hand rub, compliance rates can reach 80% (Alshehari et al. 2018). A hand hygiene compliance level of 60% is associated with a lower incidence of hospital-acquired infections (Mouajou et al. 2022). Other safety programs, such as sharps-safe disposal programs, showed increases in practitioner safety, with a 70% decline in injury rates in one hospital (Gershon et al. 1999).

In the veterinary field, there is also evidence that workplace culture and procedures significantly reduce the odds of injury. In a series of interviews conducted with veterinarians across the United Kingdom, a zoo veterinarian commented that "the risk of injury is negligible to non-existent because of the way we (work)" (O'Connor 2019). Contrastingly, a majority (60%) of large-animal veterinarians in this study expect to be injured at work, and four out of five have felt pressured to work in unsafe conditions. Clearly, the workplace culture can have a dramatic impact on safety. Given the high injury rate in practices, workplace safety deserves further attention.

PROFESSIONAL MISTAKES

Veterinary medicine is practiced by human beings, who, despite a professional tendency for perfectionism, are not perfect (Holden 2020). In one study, 74% of veterinarians acknowledged one or more medical errors in the previous 12 months (Rood and Pate 2019). Fortunately, medical errors are rare and usually not serious. A record review of the veterinary teaching hospital at Cornell University showed that for every 1,000 patients, there were an average of 5.3 medical errors or 0.53%. Over half of the mistakes were drug miscalculations (54%). The majority of errors (65.2%) either never reached the patient or did not cause any adverse event. Even when harm was caused, it was temporary in almost all patients (91.8%; Wallis et al. 2019).

Despite the rarity of medical errors and low likelihood of harm to patients, the psychological impacts on the practitioner can be profound (Kogan et al. 2018). Even when medical errors had no impact on patients; at least a quarter of veterinarians reported losing confidence in their ability as a doctor, a decrease in job satisfaction, and burnout. These feelings persisted despite the majority of vets receiving support and empathy from both their colleagues and supervisors. Negative impacts from near misses lasted for more than a week for over one-third of veterinarians polled, and 10% of those who experienced a near miss began to question their career choice (Kogan et al. 2018). Together, these two studies paint a picture of a career in which mistakes are uncommon and rarely have long-term negative effects on patients, yet still carry a significant emotional toll.

In Story 6.1, a veterinarian recounts a professional mistake. After an accident left a patient with burns, the veterinarian took several steps to address the situation. They disclosed the mistake to both the client and their leadership. They also debriefed with her technicians. These debriefing sessions provide both emotional support after a mistake and an opportunity for analysis, and, if appropriate, changes to policy and the procedure. These actions can help medical professionals to handle the emotional impacts of a mistake better (Robertson and Long 2018). It is also worth considering that if you cultivate an environment in which folks are confident they will be supported when disclosing an error, they will be more likely to do so.

MORAL DILEMMAS AND DISTRESS

In veterinary medicine, moral dilemmas arise that involve balancing professional obligations and personal values. These are also commonly referred to as ethical dilemmas and distress. For example, clients may refuse to agree to recommended treatment because of financial constraints, and the veterinarian must balance their obligation to the animal patient against the demands of the human client or requirements imposed on them by their employer. Moral distress results from exposure to moral dilemmas when the practitioner knows what the right thing is to do, but they are prevented from doing it. The nature of medicine means that veterinarians will inevitably encounter morally distressing situations. Less than 2% of a sample of 889 veterinarians in North America reported that they had *never* been asked to do something

STORY 6.1 PROFESSIONAL MISTAKES

I was doing a dental on a rabbit. At the time, I had been boarded as an exotics specialist for about three years. I had done dozens of these procedures, so it felt fairly routine. The rabbit was on a mask, and my technician was monitoring anesthesia.

I was in the middle of surgically addressing an abscess when I hit a bigger blood vessel. This is a fairly common complication of the procedure and usually is more annoying than dangerous. I decided to use a hand cautery wand. I was being really careful, but my hand slipped and I got too close to the mask. It caught fire, as did my patient's face. I immediately pulled the mask off and threw it into the sink, and my tech put a towel on the rabbit's head.

There was an immediate moment of utter panic. The mask was still actively on fire as I ran it over to the sink. It didn't even occur to me to turn off the oxygen, which should have been my first move. Once I knew the patient was alive and the fire was out, I had to force myself to breathe and think, but a thousand thoughts and feelings were running through my head all at the same time. Do I wake the patient up and not finish the procedure? Do I need to intubate? Do I need to get the hospital admin involved? How do I talk to the owner? All the questions came at the same time, and of course, the overwhelming embarrassment and shame that I had let this happen. After a moment, the doctor part of my brain took over, and I just put one foot in front of the other, so to speak.

I turned off the gas and assessed the damage. The burns were covering her nasal planum, lips, and the right side of her nose, so I was immediately very concerned about the nasal damage and respiratory compromise, but we still needed to finish the surgery. I remember my heart was pounding so hard. I felt completely flooded with adrenaline. I finished the surgery as quickly as I could. I don't think I've ever sutured that fast. I recovered the rabbit in oxygen, and thank god she was fairly stable.

I called my boss first. I wanted to touch base with her before I called the owner. She came down with some other people in admin to discuss what happened. She was honestly a bit shocked that I was ready to call the client. She thought, when I called her, that I was too shaken, and I wanted her to do it. In reality, I just wanted to make sure it was okay to say the hospital would pay for the care. We discussed what I would say to the client and that the hospital would cover any charges for the burns.

I called the client, and she was honestly lovely. She was a retired nurse. I explained what happened and that her rabbit was okay and that we would be treating the burns. Her reply was "Oh we see this happen in human medicine all the time. Don't worry. Are you ok?"

She could have berated me. Instead, she was so kind and empathetic. So were my colleagues. Everyone was just really supportive. Had this happened in some of the previous places I worked, it would have been very different, especially if it had happened during my residency. If I had an error like that there, I would have been lectured and scolded and would not have gotten any support in talking to the owner.

Don't get me wrong, even with the support, it still wasn't easy. The techs and I sat down that evening and talked about what happened. When I went home that night, I was completely mentally and physically drained. It was pretty difficult to get up and go to work the next morning, too. I felt like I was in a fog that whole day. For days, I had a lot of guilt that I could have burned down the ward and hurt my techs. It's three years later, and I still remember there were eight patients on that ward, and I could have killed them all with one slip of my hand. For weeks, I had nightmares about the ward burning down. However, the support I received from the owner and my colleagues helped me be kinder to myself. I still couldn't stop thinking about it for weeks, but their support helped me think it through logically and made me feel less guilty.

Table 6.1 Common moral dilemmas in practice.

- Compromising patient care due to financial limitations
- Being asked to provide treatment that the practitioner does not believe is in the patient's best interest or may be futile
- Balancing the desires and welfare of the client with the welfare of the patient
- Being asked to do things outside of the practitioner's skillset
- Being asked to perform surgical procedures that are cosmetic or based on convenience rather than medical need
- Disclosing medical errors
- Working with colleagues who are providing incompetent or unethical care
- Performing euthanasias that are motivated by client convenience or financial limitations
- Making decisions around reporting and intervening in suspected animal abuse.

Source: Adapted From Jurney (2022).

that felt wrong in their clinical practice (Moses et al. 2018). Not only is the experience nearly universal, it also occurs frequently. More than half of veterinarians reported facing a moral dilemma at least once a day (Kipperman et al. 2017). A list of common moral dilemmas is available in Table 6.1.

Over time, moral distress can negatively impact mental health and job satisfaction, leading to increased employee turnover (Chun et al. 2019; Jurney and Kipperman 2022). In one study, 77% of veterinarians identified ethical conflicts as a moderate or primary contributor to their level of burnout (Kipperman et al. 2017).

Factors Contributing to the Experience of Moral Distress

Veterinary professionals experience moral dilemmas and distress to varying degrees. Factors that make one susceptible to moral stress encompass demographic, environmental, and personality-based risk factors.

Demographically, female and younger veterinarians tend to encounter a higher frequency of serious psychological distress and can perceive moral dilemmas as more stressful than their counterparts (Nett et al. 2015; Kipperman et al. 2018). This pattern echoes broader population-level trends in which young people and women report higher rates of mental health concerns (SAMHSA 2024), suggesting this is not unique to veterinary medicine.

The experience of empathy may also contribute to demographic risk. Female veterinarians and veterinary students have been shown to have higher levels of empathy toward animals and greater concern for their welfare compared to male peers, which may predispose them to heightened ethical distress (Colombo et al. 2017; Paul and Podberscek 2000). Empathy also appears to shift with age and clinical exposure. With experience, veterinarians tend to develop stronger empathy for clients, which can soften conflict when patient care is constrained by finances or owner decisions (Springer et al. 2021). A less experienced clinician may view the situation primarily through the lens of the animal's needs and experience frustration or resentment toward the client. Over time, the ability to empathize with both parties can reduce the adversarial tone of ethical dilemmas and lessen their emotional impact. Experience, in this way, moderates the negative emotional toll of morally stressful events (Crane et al. 2015).

Beyond empathy, other personality factors play an important role. Perfectionism has been consistently identified as a trait that increases vulnerability to moral stressors in veterinarians (Crane et al. 2015). In veterinary populations, perfectionism is strongly associated with neurotic personality traits (Holden 2020), and neuroticism has been linked to more intense negative psychological responses to moral distress in the medical field (Kok et al. 2023). Individuals high in perfectionism or neuroticism are therefore more likely to internalize moral conflict, ruminate, and experience guilt or self-blame when they feel unable to provide ideal care (Crane et al. 2015; Smith et al. 2022; Holden 2020).

Occupational factors further shape risk. Greater working hours and workload intensity increase the stress response to moral conflict (Crane et al. 2015), mirroring trends in human healthcare where work–life conflict is a predictor of moral distress (Kok 2023). Job role also matters. Veterinary nurses and technicians appear particularly vulnerable, especially when required to perform treatments they perceive as futile or harmful (Quain et al. 2021; Peterson 2025). The impact of moral stressors is intensified in a companion-animal practice, where the cultural shift toward viewing pets as family members increases the emotional stakes for staff (Quain et al. 2021; Ouedraogo et al. 2021).

Feelings of inadequacy or lack of confidence in navigating ethical challenges also correlate with higher distress among nurses and technicians, which opens the door for a potential intervention (Quain et al. 2021). Quain (2021) found that clinicians who feel more competent in addressing ethical and moral conflicts report less distress, suggesting that education in conflict resolution, ethics, and communication may offer a protective pathway. Strengthening these skills may help veterinary teams navigate ethically complex cases with greater clarity, confidence, and emotional resilience.

Responding to Moral Distress

The most common moral dilemma reported by small-animal veterinarians is that client economic limitations affect their ability to practice (Kipperman et al. 2017). When asked how they might address this limitation, the majority of veterinarians agreed that greater adoption of pet insurance by their clients would help resolve this dilemma. However, only 23% of these veterinarians routinely discuss pet insurance with pet owners (Kipperman et al. 2017). When asked why they are not implementing this solution, veterinarians reported a lack of time as a barrier and disbelief that their clients would listen. It is essential to consider ways to respond to moral distress and implement them whenever practical.

Dealing with complex, morally distressing situations takes time, which is a rare commodity in veterinary practice (Fawcett and Mullan 2018; Rushton 2016). A practitioner who has appointments booked every 20 minutes doesn't have time to ponder and research thoughtful solutions, but objective analysis and precise action plans have both been shown to decrease moral stress (Morris 2012; Rushton 2016; Carse et al. 2017). Knowing that certain moral dilemmas are common in veterinary medicine, practitioners can benefit from making advance preparations. One important step is to identify your moral values. A number of value exercises can be found online, such as those on Brené Brown's website (https://brenebrown.com/resources/living-into-our-values/). Being familiar with your values enables you to recognize morally distressing situations and respond in ways that align with your personal moral code.

After this work is done, you can consider common clinical scenarios discussed in Table 6.1 and how best to mitigate them while staying true to your values. For the above example about pet insurance, practice workflows could be developed, such as adding a question on client check-in paperwork about pet insurance. Front desk staff can offer insurance pamphlets or explain how their bill could be decreased if they had insurance. In these brief actions, the client is being made aware of pet insurance and the team takes steps to mitigate a significant cause of distress before it becomes an issue. Practitioners can also craft a policy outlining the steps to follow when faced with a client who cannot afford care. By doing all of this work in advance, you will reduce the time and effort required in the moment, when emotions are running high and empower employees to act quickly when situations arise.

Discussing difficult situations in team meetings also reduces moral distress in healthcare settings (Vaclavik et al., 2018; Krautscheid et al., 2020). Team meetings enable collective planning for similar situations in the future, which empowers employees to exercise their moral agency and take action in the workplace. Working in an environment where employees feel supported in making moral decisions without fear of negative consequences significantly reduces the risk of moral distress (Carse et al. 2017). Lower levels of workplace autonomy, as reported by female-identified veterinarians and support staff, may also be associated with greater moral distress (Wallace 2019). The contributions of workplace culture to mental health will be discussed at length in Chapter 7.

Finally, physical and emotional self-care are crucial to fostering moral resilience (Shapiro et al. 2019; Volk et al. 2020). Practicing mindfulness, maintaining a healthy diet, and getting enough sleep are not going to alleviate distress related to a client's request for convenience euthanasia. However, self-care practices promote effective stress management, both physically and mentally. Simply put, no one will perform well in a complicated and emotional situation when they are exhausted, dehydrated, and holding their bladder. Self-care and cognitive skills will be discussed in detail in Chapter 10.

COMPASSION FATIGUE, SECONDARY TRAUMATIC STRESS, AND POSTTRAUMATIC STRESS DISORDER

Compassion fatigue (CF) was first defined by Figley (1995) as a state of biological, psychological, and social exhaustion that develops from prolonged engagement in compassionately helping others who are suffering or traumatized. In Figley's original conceptualization, compassion fatigue was considered synonymous with secondary traumatic stress (STS), a construct first described in therapists who developed trauma-like symptoms after repeatedly hearing clients describe violent or distressing events (Figley 1995).

As the field evolved, Stamm introduced the Professional Quality of Life scale (ProQOL), which remains the most widely used tool for assessing compassion fatigue in veterinary settings (Noe et al. 2024). The ProQOL expanded the definition of compassion fatigue by dividing it into two measurable components, burnout and secondary traumatic stress, and included a separate measure of compassion satisfaction (Stamm 2010). Compassion satisfaction (CS) reflects the pleasure and meaning derived from helping others, whereas burnout and STS capture the emotional costs of caregiving. As such, in the literature, rates of compassion fatigue are reported as separate CS, STS, and burnout scores. As Chapter 9 examines burnout in detail, the discussion here focuses on STS and its relationship to posttraumatic stress disorder (PTSD).

Secondary Traumatic Stress (STS)

STS describes trauma-like symptoms that arise from indirect exposure to distressing events, typically through caregiving or repeated exposure to suffering (Stamm 2010). The ProQOL measures symptoms such as intrusive thoughts, nightmares, hyperarousal, avoidance, emotional numbing, concentration difficulties, and sleep disruption. In veterinary workplaces, clinicians and staff describe being "haunted" by distressing cases, withdrawing from emotional interactions at work, avoiding euthanasia or certain clients, or replaying cases after hours (Hayes et al. 2020; Ouedraogo et al. 2021). These patterns have been documented among veterinary emergency and critical care teams, shelter and animal control staff, and general practice clinicians (Hayes et al. 2020; Bennett and Rohlf 2005; Kogan et al. 2021). Table 6.2 summarizes ProQOL findings reported in several veterinary studies. Across studies of veterinary professionals, mean ProQOL scores typically fall within moderate ranges for CS, burnout, and STS. However, in shelter workers, high STS scores occur in more than 90% of participants. In contrast, CS generally remains moderate to high across studies. Taken together, these findings show that veterinary medicine is demanding and emotionally taxing for many professionals, yet most still derive a strong sense of purpose and fulfillment from their work.

STS in clinical veterinary practice is closely linked to repeated exposure to emotionally distressing events. Performing euthanasia and witnessing animal suffering are consistently associated with higher STS scores among clinical veterinarians (Ouedraogo et al. 2021). Client-related challenges, including delivering bad news and navigating confrontational or highly emotional interactions, further increase risk (Rohlf et al. 2022). Moral distress also plays a substantial role, particularly when financial limitations or client preferences prevent clinicians from providing ideal care, or when euthanasia is pursued under constrained circumstances (Kogan and Rishniw 2023). The cumulative nature of these clinical stressors is also evident: A greater number of highly distressing cases are correlated with elevated trauma-related symptoms, even when single events are not severe (Kramper et al. 2023). These patterns are especially pronounced in emergency

Table 6.2 ProQol scores across veterinary studies.

Study	Population	Sample size (*n*)	Compassion satisfaction	Burnout	Secondary Traumatic Stress
Smith (2016)	Veterinary nurses, UK	992	99% moderate / high CS	92.% moderate / high risk	68.1% moderate / high risk
Ouedraogo et al. (2021)	Canadian veterinary technicians	401	35.5% low	50.2% high	58.9% high
Perret et al. (2020)	Veterinarians, Canada	1274	28.1% low / 40.3% moderate / 31.6% high	22.3% low / 35.6% moderate / 41.7% high	3.8% low / 30.8% moderate / 65.4% high
Scotney et al. (2019)	Mixed animal-care, majority vet practice	229	Mean 39.2 (moderate)	Mean 24.8 (moderate)	Mean 24.6 (moderate)
Alwood et al. (2024)*	ER & specialty hospital staff, US	34	mean 37.5 (moderate)	Mean ~24.8 (moderate)	Mean ~24.9 (moderate)
Wolf et al. (2024)	Shelter staff, US	243	11.5% low / 39.1% moderate / 49.4% high	14.4% low / 32.1% moderate / 53.5% high	0.8% low / 8.2% moderate / 90.9% high

Using Stamm's standard ProQOL cutoffs on the 10–50 scale, scores of 22 or below fall into the low range, 23–41 indicate moderate concern, and scores of 42 or higher are considered high. Across studies reporting categorical results, a substantial portion of participants fell in the moderate range for burnout and secondary traumatic stress, with some cohorts showing notably elevated proportions in the high range. Comparisons should note that Ouedraogo et al. (2021) used percentile-based thresholds (top 25%) rather than fixed ProQOL cutoffs, which can inflate the proportion classified as "high" relative to studies using the standard scoring system.

*Alwood et al. (2024) reported separate baseline ProQOL scores for intervention and control groups prior to a resilience-building program. Because the purpose of this table is to compare pre-intervention ProQOL values across studies, the two baseline groups were combined into a single weighted mean to represent the overall sample.

and critical care settings, where sudden loss, frequent euthanasia, and high-stakes decision-making are common (Scotney et al. 2015). Taken together, the literature demonstrates that secondary traumatic stress in clinical practice arises not only from acute traumatic events but also from the repeated emotional demands inherent to everyday veterinary work.

Posttraumatic Stress Disorder

Although STS shares symptom features with PTSD, they are not the same. PTSD is defined in the *Diagnostic and Statistical Manual of Mental Disorders (DSM)* and requires meeting multiple symptom clusters as well as functional impairment. Critically, Criterion A requires exposure to "actual or threatened death, serious injury, or sexual violence" (American Psychiatric Association, 2022, p. 301) and applies only to events involving human victims. Because veterinary professionals care for animals, not humans, many of the most distressing clinical experiences would not technically qualify as a traumatic event per the DSM. As a result, PTSD prevalence in veterinarians appears low when measured by the defined criteria. For example, Penix et al. (2019) reported that approximately 5% of US military veterinary professionals scored at risk of PTSD.

The restrictive definition of PTSD leaves room for potential underdiagnosis in the veterinary population. Kramper et al. (2023) provide a clear illustration of this issue. When PTSD was assessed using traditional, strict DSM definitions, only 21.1% of veterinarians reported a Criterion A trauma at work, most commonly injuries to themselves or staff or threats of violence from clients. When the authors expanded Criterion A to include traumatic events involving animals, the proportion nearly doubled to 39.3% (Kramper et al., 2023). However, exposure to a traumatic event does not guarantee development of symptoms and PTSD remained relatively uncommon: 3.6% (traditional criteria) and 13.9% (expanded criteria) screened positive. These rates are similar to what is reported by physicians (14.8%; Jacob Sendler et al. 2016). The study also demonstrated that repeated exposure was associated with higher symptom likelihood, highlighting the cumulative nature of traumatic stress in veterinary work.

Protective Factors and Management Strategies

Although emotionally difficult cases are unavoidable in veterinary medicine, several factors help buffer the impact of compassion fatigue, STS, and PTSD. Support from colleagues, family, and supervisors consistently protects against trauma-related symptoms, and clinicians who feel psychologically safe at work report fewer intrusive thoughts and faster recovery (Thabet and Vostanis 2017). Individual skills such as emotional regulation, reflective processing, and self-compassion further lower vulnerability. Among animal care workers, emotional intelligence and self-compassion show a moderate negative relationship with STS, suggesting these capacities can be strengthened over time (Monaghan et al. 2024). Mindfulness-based interventions also reduce distress and improve sleep in healthcare teams (Kim et al. 2022). These skills are covered in more detail in Chapter 10.

When symptoms persist, trauma-informed psychological treatments such as trauma-focused cognitive behavioral therapy and EMDR are effective for reducing PTSD symptoms (Kim et al. 2022).

Within organizational structure, debriefs after potentially traumatic events may also be helpful. In a recent survey of veterinarians, high-quality debriefings after adverse medical events were associated with greater psychological safety, higher job fulfilment, increased work engagement, and reduced burnout, even when controlling for work setting and debriefing frequency (Kogan and Rishniw 2023). Participants described feeling supported, heard, and more hopeful about improvement. However, poorly executed debriefings – those that felt judgmental or emotionally unsafe – were associated with greater emotional exhaustion, anxiety, and frustration (Devilly and

Cotton 2003; Kogan and Rishniw 2023). Debriefings, therefore, appear protective only when they are structured, blame-free, and facilitated by trained leaders focused on learning rather than fault.

DISASTER RESPONSE

Veterinary professionals have an essential role to play in many emergencies, ranging from natural disasters to public health emergencies. Unfortunately, this can take a toll. 51% of veterinary workers involved in disaster response report negative mental health impacts both during and six months after the disaster (see Figure 6.1; Vroegindewey and Kertis 2021). Emergency situations present not only practical challenges, such as access to equipment and appropriate facilities, but also greater exposure to distressing circumstances. Furthermore, veterinary professionals may be required to perform tasks like depopulation, which can result in moral injury as well as STS (Galles 2023).

In Story 6.2, we see the story of a mixed-animal vet who was involved in the foot and mouth outbreak. She details how she was exposed to not only STS in witnessing the stress of the farmers but also primary stress from her role in the depopulation. Direct participation in a lethal act that causes moral injury, such as this vet having to perform multiple euthanasias outside of standard ethical guidelines, puts the practitioner at risk for a variant of PTSD called perpetration-induced traumatic stress (PITS). Beginning with the study of Vietnam War veterans, it has been recognized that direct participation in lethal action significantly increases the chance of PTSD (Whiting and Marion 2011). PITS has been recognized as a risk in a number of animal-related fields, including lab animal and shelter medicine (Bennett and Rohlf 2005).

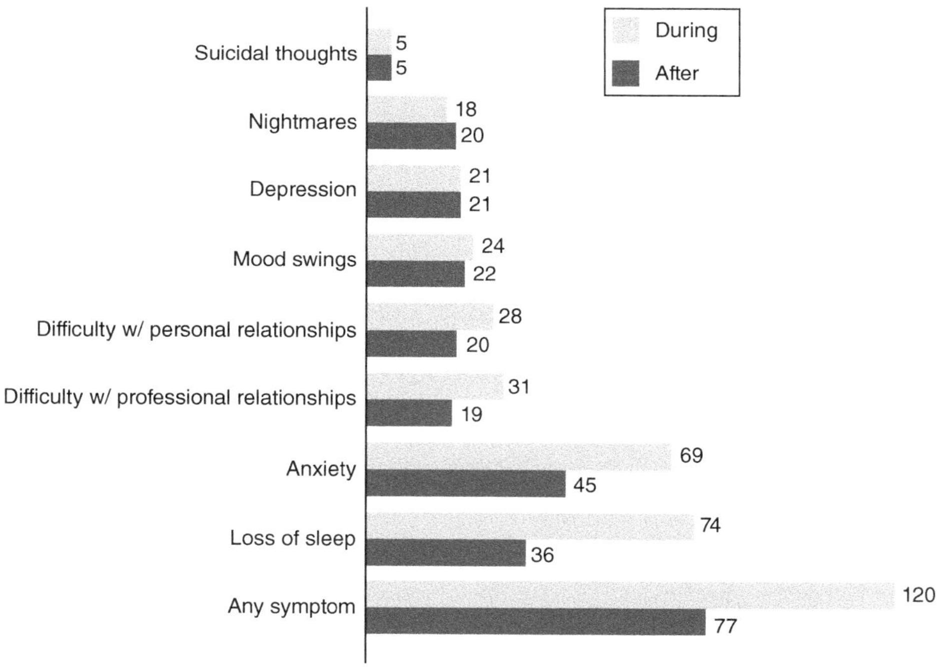

FIGURE 6.1 The numbers of reported behavioral health issues experienced during the disaster response and six months after the disaster response by symptom type ($n = 240$). This figure/material is reproduced with permission from the author and the Australian Government Department of Home Affairs 2025. The article was first printed in the Australian *Journal of Emergency Management*, 36(3):78-84, July 2021. Current and past issues of the journal are available at Australian Journal of Emergency Management | AJEM (Vroegindewey and Kertis (2021).

STORY 6.2 DISASTER RESPONSE

I was 23 years old, just six months out of vet school when it happened. I was a mixed animal practitioner in Devon, which is in the southwest corner of the United Kingdom. One Thursday night, I was out at one of the farms pulling calves. The cow was from a rare line of Devon cattle and had twins that were all tangled up. The farmer and I were making small talk as I was untangling them, and he mentioned that his neighbor had something weird going on with his cows. At the time, I thought nothing of it.

The next day was my day off. My boss called me in a bit of a panic. I needed to get back to the office asap. That neighboring farm had foot and mouth. It was, in fact, one of the very first farms to get identified. And I had been next door the night before, so I was contaminated.

Being one of the only vets contaminated, I was then tasked with the inspections. I was the one who had to start the culling. Two days after I pulled those calves, I had to cull them and the entire herd.

Very quickly, it became apparent that there was no possible way to follow any normal protocol. The strict ethical guidelines that had been drilled into my head on welfare during slaughter were out the window. I knew we were doing the best we could with the tools available, but I also knew that under other circumstances, we would have been charged with negligence.

Initially, the government required us to burn the bodies. That was particularly frustrating because there was evidence from the last outbreak that fire actually could spread the disease. So we were forced to do something we knew wasn't a good idea. Eventually, the volume was overwhelming, and the army was sent in. They were supposed to help with the culling, but so many of those soldiers couldn't handle it. They were trained to kill in a conflict, but this was different. So that job largely fell on the vets. And it went on for months. Three to four months of heavy-duty culling. We culled 50% of the farms in our practice; more than 200 farms. And the ones that did survive had constant problems with supplies; they couldn't move milk trucks and feed trucks. Farmers were desperate. They would threaten the government vets who wanted to come on their property with guns. It was a nightmare.

One farm I went to, I was really concerned about the farmer. I had the police remove his guns because I worried he was going to hurt himself or someone else. The next day, my boss called with the terrible news that the farmer had taken his life. Years later, I still feel responsible for his death.

I don't think I've ever fully recovered from it. It's been more than 20 years, and I still lose sleep over it.

Specific interventions for PITS have yet to be validated. When the COVID-19 pandemic caused supply chain failures necessitating the depopulation of swine in North America, the psychological impacts of disaster response was mitigated by sleep and socialization with friends and family (Baysinger and Kogan 2022). Presumably, social support helps balance out one of the top stressors of depopulation: the perception of the actions by others (Baysinger and Kogan 2022). Without full context of the circumstances, veterinary professionals tasked with these difficult duties can face intense scrutiny from the general public, as well as their colleagues, family, and friends. However, through socializing, these practitioners can reconnect with these communities and, hopefully, increase understanding and access support.

The public health authorities in Story 6.2 made decisions about body disposal directly against the advice of veterinarians, and the veterinarians were still required to follow those orders. When people with material knowledge are silenced or excluded from decisions, it is called epistemic injustice (Byskov 2021). Epistemic injustice, along with bearing witness to the trauma of animals and people directly impacted by the emergency, was found to be associated with the greatest experiences of psychological distress in veterinarians responding to a Mycoplasma bovis outbreak in New Zealand in 2018 (Doolan-Noble et al. 2023). We can see the impact of bearing witness on the young veterinarian in Story 6.2, as she discusses the impacts on the farm community, as well as her lingering feelings of guilt after a farmer's suicide.

Despite the numerous difficulties that may be encountered, there are potential benefits from disaster response. Individuals involved in disaster response can report that the experiences are rewarding and leave them with increased self-esteem, compassion, and a stronger connection to their communities (Brooks 2018). The key is a focus on resilience and subsequent posttraumatic growth. In a review examining resilience and posttraumatic growth in disaster-exposed organizations, three areas were found to be important: appropriate training for job roles, social support, and coping mechanisms (Brooks 2018). Individuals who are specifically prepared for their roles and tasks in a disaster and feel some level of mastery and competence in these roles have been found to have higher resilience and are less likely to have lasting psychological impacts postdisaster (Brooks 2018). While some veterinarians involved in disasters, such as those deployed through government agencies like the National Veterinary Response Team, may have access to disaster-specific training, it is not commonplace. Given the nature of disasters and response, veterinarians without the training may also be called to assist. In this instance, the presence of robust social support, as well as encouragement toward proactive coping, is essential in mitigating the psychological impacts of disaster response (Brooks 2018).

REFERENCES

Alshehari, A.A., Park, S., and Rashid, H. (2018). Strategies to improve hand hygiene compliance among healthcare workers in adult intensive care units: a mini systematic review. *Journal of Hospital Infection* 100 (2): 152–158.

Alwood, A.J., Caylor, K.B., Delany, A., Crowley, A. and Moffett, J.E. (2024). The positive impact of daily well-being practices on individual veterinary workers' professional quality of life, *Frontiers in Veterinary Science* 11: 1381090.

American Psychiatric Association (2022). *Diagnostic and Statistical Manual of Mental Disorders* (5th ed., text rev.; DSM-5-TR). American Psychiatric Publishing.

American Veterinary Medical Association (AVMA). (2021). Cyberbullying Survey Results 2014/2021. Unpublished internal presentation, presented by Laura Pikel, 16 September 2021.

American Veterinary Medical Association (AVMA). (2022). Client Interactions & Cyberbullying Survey Results. Unpublished internal presentation, presented by Laura Pikel, 18 November 2022.

Baysinger, A. and Kogan, L.R. (2022). Mental health impact of mass depopulation of swine on veterinarians during COVID-19 infrastructure breakdown. *Frontiers in Veterinary Science* 9: 842585.

Bennett, P. and Rohlf, V. (2005). Perpetration-induced traumatic stress in persons who euthanize nonhuman animals in surgeries, animal shelters, and laboratories. *Society and Animals* 13 (3): 201–220.

Brooks, S.K., Amlôt, R., Rubin, G.J., and Greenberg, N. (2018). Psychological resilience and post-traumatic growth in disaster-exposed organisations: overview of the literature. *Journal of the Royal Army Medical Corps* https://doi.org/10.1136/jramc-2017-000876.

Bryce, A.R., Rossi, T.A., Tansey, C. et al. (2019). Effect of client complaints on small animal veterinary internists. *Journal of Small Animal Practice* 60 (3): 167–172.

Byskov, M.F. (2021). What makes epistemic injustice an "injustice"? *Journal of Social Philosophy* 52 (1): 114–131.

Cake, M.A., Bell, M.A., Bickley, N., and Bartram, D.J. (2015). The life of meaning: a model of the positive contributions to well-being from veterinary work. *Journal of Veterinary Medical Education* 42 (3): 184–193.

Carse, E., Lantos, J., Rushton, C., and Sinclair, S. (2017). Moral distress in healthcare: causes, consequences, and proposed solutions. *Clinical Ethics* 12 (1): 18–25.

Christian, K. and Ohio, C. (2020). Finding Confidence in Conflict: How to Negotiate Anything and Live your Best Life. Columbus, Ohio: American Negotiation Institute. pg. 14

Chuai, Y. and Zhao, J. (2022). Anger can make fake news viral online. *Frontiers in Physics* 10: 970174.

Chun, M.S., Joo, S., and Jung, Y. (2019). Veterinary ethical issues and stressfulness of ethical dilemmas of Korean veterinarians. In: *Sustainable Governance and Management of Food Systems: Ethical Perspectives*, 193–202. Wageningen Academic Publishers.

Colombo, E.S., Crippa, F., Calderari, T., and Prato-Previde, E. (2017). Empathy toward animals and people: the role of gender and length of service in a sample of Italian veterinarians. *Journal of Veterinary Behavior* 17: 32–37.

Crane, M.F., Phillips, J.K., and Karin, E. (2015). Trait perfectionism strengthens the negative effects of moral stressors occurring in veterinary practice. *Australian Veterinary Journal* 93 (10): 354–360.

Devilly, G.J. and Cotton, P. (2003). Psychological debriefing and the prevention of posttraumatic stress. *Australian Psychologist* 38 (2): 82–87.

Doolan-Noble, F., Noller, G., Jaye, C., and Bryan, M. (2023). Moral distress in rural veterinarians as an outcome of the Mycoplasma bovis incursion in southern New Zealand. *New Zealand Veterinary Journal* 71 (3): 116–127.

Fan, R., Xu, K., and Zhao, J. (2018). An agent-based model for emotion contagion and competition in online social media. *Physica A: Statistical Mechanics and its Applications* 495: 245–259.

Fawcett, A. and Mullan, S. (2018). Managing moral distress in practice. *In Practice* 40 (1): 34–36.

Figley, C.R. (1995). *Compassion Fatigue as Secondary Traumatic Stress Disorder: An Overview. Compassion Fatigue*. New York: Brunner/Maze.

Galles, B. (2023). A literature review of the psychosocial impacts on livestock producers and veterinary responders involved with depopulation during and after an animal health emergency. *Capstone Experience: Master of Public Health* 263.

Gershon, R.R., Pearse, L., Grimes, M. et al. (1999). The impact of multifocused interventions on sharps injury rates at an acute-care hospital. *Infection Control & Hospital Epidemiology* 20 (12): 806–811.

Hayes, G.M., LaLonde-Paul, D.F., Perret, J.L. et al. (2020). Investigation of burnout syndrome and job-related risk factors in veterinary technicians in specialty teaching hospitals: a multicenter cross-sectional study. *Journal of Veterinary Emergency and Critical Care* 30 (1): 18–27.

Hinduja, S. and Patchin, J.W. (2014). *Bullying Beyond the Schoolyard: Preventing and Responding to Cyberbullying*. Corwin Press.

Holden, C.L. (2020). Characteristics of veterinary students: perfectionism, personality factors, and resilience. *Journal of Veterinary Medical Education* 47 (4): 488–496.

Irwin, A., Silver-MacMahon, H., and Wilcke, S. (2022). Consequences and coping: investigating client, co-worker and senior colleague incivility within veterinary practice. *Veterinary Record* 191 (7).

Jacob Sendler, D., Rutkowska, A., and Makara-Studzinska, M. (2016). How the exposure to trauma has hindered physicians' capacity to heal: prevalence of PTSD among healthcare workers. *The European Journal of Psychiatry* 30 (4): 321–334.

Jurney, C. and Kipperman, B. (2022). Moral stress. In: *Ethics in Veterinary Practice: Balancing Conflicting Interests*, 460–480.

Kim, J., Chesworth, B., Franchino-Olsen, H., and Macy, R.J. (2022). A scoping review of vicarious trauma interventions for service providers working with people who have experienced traumatic events. *Trauma, Violence & Abuse* 23 (5): 1437–1460.

Kipperman, B.S., Kass, P.H., and Rishniw, M. (2017). Factors that influence small animal veterinarians' opinions and actions regarding cost of care and effects of economic limitations on patient care and outcome and professional career satisfaction and burnout. *Journal of the American Veterinary Medical Association* 250 (7): 785–794.

Kipperman, B., Morris, P., and Rollin, B. (2018). Ethical dilemmas encountered by small animal veterinarians: characterisation, responses, consequences and beliefs regarding euthanasia. *Veterinary Record* 182 (19): 548–548.

Kogan, L.R., Rishniw, M., Hellyer, P.W., and Schoenfeld-Tacher, R.M. (2018). Veterinarians' experiences with near misses and adverse events. *Journal of the American Veterinary Medical Association* 252 (5): 586–595.

Kogan, L.R. and Rishniw, M. (2023). Veterinarians and moral distress. *Journal of the American Veterinary Medical Association* 261 (5): 1–7.

Kok, N., Van Gurp, J., Van Der Hoeven, J.G. et al. (2023). Complex interplay between moral distress and other risk factors of burnout in ICU professionals: findings from a cross-sectional survey study. *BMJ Quality & Safety* 32 (4): 225–234.

Kramper, S., Crosby, E.S., Waitz-Kudla, S.N. et al. (2023). Highly stressful events and posttraumatic stress disorder symptoms among veterinary professionals: Prevalence and associations with mental health and job-related outcomes. *Psychological trauma: theory, research, practice, and policy* 15 (S2): S275.

Krautscheid, L., Caine, R., and Thompson, S. (2020). Moral distress consultation rounds: fostering ethical resilience in clinical teams. *Journal of Nursing Management* 28 (7): 1625–1634.

Lotfinejad, N., Peters, A., Tartari, E. et al. (2021). Hand hygiene in health care: 20 years of ongoing advances and perspectives. *The Lancet Infectious Diseases* 21 (8): e209–e221.

Morris, P. (2012). Coping with euthanasia: Emotion-management strategies. In: *Blue Juice: Euthanasia in Veterinary Medicine*, 136–169. Philadelphia, PA: Temple University Press.

Moses, L., Malowney, M.J., and Wesley Boyd, J. (2018). Ethical conflict and moral distress in veterinary practice: A survey of North American veterinarians. *Journal of veterinary internal medicine* 32 (6): 2115–2122.

Monaghan, E., Berry, L., and Walker, C. (2024). Self-compassion and emotional intelligence as predictors of secondary traumatic stress in animal-care workers. *Veterinary Sciences* 11 (1): 22.

Moore, I.C., Coe, J.B., Adams, C.L. et al. (2015). Exploring the impact of toxic attitudes and a toxic environment on the veterinary healthcare team. *Frontiers in Veterinary Science* 2: 78.

Mouajou, V., Adams, K., DeLisle, G., and Quach, C. (2022). Hand hygiene compliance in the prevention of hospital-acquired infections: a systematic review. *Journal of Hospital Infection* 119: 33–48.

Nett, R.J., Witte, T.K., Holzbauer, S.M. et al. (2015). Risk factors for suicide, attitudes toward mental illness, and practice-related stressors among US veterinarians. *Journal of the American Veterinary Medical Association* 247 (8): 945–955.

Noe, M.T.N., Baysal, Y., Masserey, A. et al. (2024). Measurement of compassion fatigue in animal health care professionals: a systematic review of available instruments and their content validity. *Frontiers in Veterinary Science* 11: 1425741.

O'Connor, E. (2019). Sources of work stress in veterinary practice in the UK. *Veterinary Record* 184 (19): 588–588.

OSHA (2022). *Survey of Occupational Injuries and Illnesses Data*. U.S. Bureau of Labor Statistics https://www.bls.gov/iif/nonfatal-injuries-and-illnesses-tables.htm#summary (accessed 24 March 2024).

Ouedraogo, F.B., Lefebvre, S.L., Hansen, C.R., and Brorsen, B.W. (2021). Compassion satisfaction, burnout, and secondary traumatic stress among full-time veterinarians in the United States (2016–2018). *Journal of the American Veterinary Medical Association* 258 (11): 1259–1270.

Paul, E.S. and Podberscek, A.L. (2000). Veterinary education and students' attitudes towards animal welfare. *Veterinary Record* 146 (10): 269–272.

Penix, E.A., Adler, A.B., Britt, T.W. and Thomas, J.L. (2019) 'Behavioral health of US military veterinary personnel deployed to Afghanistan', Journal of the American Veterinary Medical Association, 254(4), pp. 520–526. doi:https://doi.org/10.2460/javma.254.4.520.

Perret, J.L., Best, C.O., Coe, J.B., Greer, A.L., Khosa, D.K. and Jones-Bitton, A. (2020). Prevalence of mental health outcomes among Canadian veterinarians. *Journal of the American Veterinary Medical Association* 256(3): 365–375.

Peterson, N.W., Foltz, K., Moses, L., and Boyd, J.W. (2025). Veterinary technicians report in a survey how futile veterinary treatments contribute to their moral distress and impact their professional and personal lives. *Journal of the American Veterinary Medical Association* 263 (4): 473–482.

Pikel, L. (2021). Cyberbullying Survey Results. Unpublished internal survey, American Veterinary Medical Association, 16 September 2021.

Pikel, L. (2022) Client Interactions & Cyberbullying Survey Results. Unpublished internal survey, American Veterinary Medical Association, 18 November 2022.

Quain, A., Mullan, S., McGreevy, P.D., and Ward, M.P. (2021). Frequency, stressfulness and type of ethically challenging situations encountered by veterinary team members during the COVID-19 pandemic. *Frontiers in Veterinary Science* 8: 647108.

Robertson, J.J. and Long, B. (2018). Suffering in silence: medical error and its impact on health care providers. *The Journal of Emergency Medicine* 54 (4): 402–409.

Robinson, D., Edwards, M., Mason, B. et al. (2019). *The 2019 Survey of the Veterinary Profession*. Brighton, UK: Institute for Employment Studies.

Rogers, C.W., Murphy, L.A., Murphy, R.A. et al. (2022). An analysis of client complaints and their effects on veterinary support staff. *Veterinary Medicine and Science* 8 (2): 925–934.

Rohlf, V.I., Bennett, P., Toukhsati, S.R., and Coleman, G.J. (2022). Compassion fatigue in animal-related professions: a systematic review. *Journal of Applied Animal Welfare Science* 25 (3): 307–329.

Rood, K.A. and Pate, M.L. (2019). Assessment of musculoskeletal injuries associated with palpation, infection control practices, and zoonotic disease risks among Utah clinical veterinarians. *Journal of Agromedicine* 24 (1): 35–45.

Russell, E., Mossop, L., Forbes, E., and Oxtoby, C. (2022). Uncovering the 'messy details' of veterinary communication: an analysis of communication problems in cases of alleged professional negligence. *Veterinary Record* 190 (3).

Rushton, C.H. (2016). Moral resilience: A capacity for navigating moral distress in critical care. *AACN Advanced Critical Care* 27 (1): 111–119.

Scotney, R.L., McLaughlin, D., and Keates, H.L. (2015). A systematic review of the effects of euthanasia and occupational stress in personnel working with animals in animal shelters, veterinary clinics, and biomedical research facilities. *Journal of the American Veterinary Medical Association* 247 (10): 1121–1130. https://doi.org/10.2460/javma.247.10.1121.

Scotney, R.L., McLaughlin, D. and Keates, H.L. (2019). An investigation of the prevalence of compassion fatigue, compassion satisfaction and burnout in those working in animal-related occupations using the Professional Quality of Life (ProQoL) Scale. *The Veterinary Nurse* 10 (5): 276–284.

Shapiro, D.E., Duquette, C., Abbott, L.M. et al. (2019). Beyond burnout: a physician wellness hierarchy designed to prioritize interventions at the systems level. *The American journal of medicine* 132 (5): 556–563.

Smith, M.M., Sherry, S.B., Ge, S.Y. et al. (2022). Multidimensional perfectionism turns 30: A review of known knowns and known unknowns. *Canadian Psychology/Psychologie Canadienne* 63 (1): 16.

Smith, N. (2016). A questionnaire based study to assess compassion fatigue in UK practising veterinary nurses. *The Veterinary Nurse* 7 (7): 418–425.

Springer, S., Sandøe, P., Grimm, H. et al. (2021). Managing conflicting ethical concerns in modern small animal practice – a comparative study of veterinarian's decision ethics in Austria, Denmark and the UK. *PLoS One* 16 (6): e0253420.

Stamm, B.H. (2010). The concise ProQOL manual. 2e. https://proqol.org/proqol-manual (accessed 3 October 2024).

Substance Abuse and Mental Health Services Administration (SAMHSA) (2024). *NSDUH data brief: Differences in mental health among males and females aged 18 or older: 2021 and 2022*. Rockville, MD: Center for Behavioral Health Statistics and Quality, SAMHSA.

Thabet, A.A. and Vostanis, P. (2017). Social support and resilience in healthcare workers exposed to trauma. *Arab Journal of Psychiatry* 28 (1): 45–54.

Vaclavik, D., Mounsey, A., and Schlumbrecht, M. (2018). Implementation of team-based moral distress rounds: effects on burnout and ethical climate. *Journal of Clinical Nursing* 27 (21–22): 4309–4317.

Volk, J.O., Schimmack, U., Strand, E.B. et al. (2020). Executive summary of the Merck animal health veterinarian wellbeing study II. *Journal of the American Veterinary Medical Association* 256 (11): 1237–1244.

Volk, J.O., Schimmack, U., Strand, E.B. et al. (2022). Executive summary of the merck animal health veterinarian well-being study III and veterinary support staff study. *Journal of the American Veterinary Medical Association* 260 (12): 1547–1553.

Vroegindewey, G. and Kertis, K. (2021). Veterinary behavioural health issues associated with disaster response. *The Australian Journal of Emergency Management* 36 (3): 78–84.

Wallace, J.E. (2019). Meaningful work and well-being: a study of the positive side of veterinary work. *Veterinary Record* 185 (18): 571–571.

Wallis, J., Fletcher, D., Bentley, A., and Ludders, J. (2019). Medical errors cause harm in veterinary hospitals. *Frontiers in Veterinary Science* 6: 12.

Whiting, T.L. and Marion, C.R. (2011). Perpetration-induced traumatic stress – a risk for veterinarians involved in the destruction of healthy animals. *The Canadian Veterinary Journal* 52 (7): 794.

Wolf, P.J., Protopopova, A., Ly, L.H., Friedmann, E. and Guenther, K.M. (2024). Measures of well-being in U.S. animal shelter staff during 2023, *Journal of Applied Shelter Veterinary Medicine* 3(1).

CHAPTER 7 Workplace Culture Well-being

Carrie Jurney, DVM, DACVIM (Neurology)[1] and Lori Kogan, PhD[2]

[1] *Not One More Vet, Inc, San Francisco, CA, USA*

[2] *Colorado State University, College of Veterinary Medicine and Biomedical Sciences, Fort Collins, CO, USA*

INTRODUCTION

In Chapter 6, we discussed some of the challenges many of us face regardless of our environment. In this chapter, we shift to the environment and discuss qualities that are directly linked to the culture of a specific workplace, and how to manage elements that can threaten your well-being.

Workplace culture is the collection of values, expectations, and practices that influence the behavior of all team members (Kogan and Rishniw 2024). More than just a list of rules, culture impacts unspoken behaviors, mindsets, and social patterns (Groysberg et al. 2018). Much research has been done around specific aspects of culture, like leadership or hours worked, and their impact on well-being. In this chapter, we will review the effect of these factors in detail. However, at the end of the day, culture is more than the sum of its parts. It is a living, breathing, and evolving influence that touches every aspect of our work life.

So, how important is workplace culture? In Chapters 2 and 10, we highlight the importance of personality and personal coping mechanisms in well-being, which, according to several authors, has the biggest impact on our well-being (Dawson and Thompson 2017; Volk et al. 2024). However, this does not negate the impact of workplace culture on our professional satisfaction and engagement. In the Merck Veterinary Wellbeing Study, workplace culture was second only to personal coping mechanisms in predicting well-being and burnout (Volk et al. 2024). Multiple studies have found the quality of the workplace culture to be key in veterinary employee retention (Hagen 2020; Kogan 2022, 2024). In the ideal scenario, a healthy workplace and a healthy team form a positive feedback loop, enhancing everyone's well-being. In this chapter, we discuss the building blocks of a healthy culture and how all team members can identify, benefit, and contribute to this dynamic.

THE JOBS DEMANDS RESOURCES MODEL

What makes some jobs more stressful than others? A popular model used to describe the interaction of job characteristics and their impact on well-being is called the Jobs Demands-Resources model (JD-R; Bakker 2023). This model emphasizes the balance between the demands of our job, or those things that require effort and have some physiologic or psychological cost, and our resources. When the demand exceeds our resources, we tend to feel stressed and burned out (Bakker 2023). In a survey of French veterinarians, workplace stressors were sorted into nine categories: negative work–home interactions, coworker issues, workload, burden of responsibility, financial issues, emotional demands, issues with clients, and feeling in danger (Andela 2020). All jobs have stressors, and the goal of a healthy culture is not to eliminate them entirely. However, a healthy work environment strives to minimize demands while also providing adequate resources.

Resources are often divided into professional resources (e.g. task autonomy – the level of control one is allowed over how a job is done, support from colleagues, and management support), and personal resources (e.g. self-efficacy – one's personal belief in their ability to accomplish a

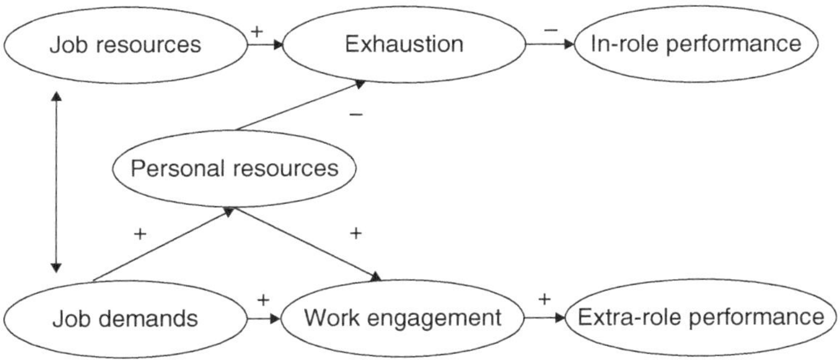

FIGURE 7.1 The extended job demands resources model (Mastenbroek, et al 2014 / with permision of John Wiley & Sons).

task, optimism, thoughtfulness, intrinsic motivation, and assertiveness) (Mastenbroek et al. 2014). The interaction between demands, resources, burnout, and engagement can be seen in Figure 7.1 (Mastenbroek 2014).

We see this play out in our field in many ways. For instance, when asked which work environment they preferred, 55% of veterinarians chose a private practice, while 12% chose a corporate practice (Kogan and Rishniw 2024). Interestingly, 46% of people who crrently work in corporate practice indicated a preference for private practice. On the one hand, much of the actual work done within corporate and private practices is similar. In this study, the ability to obtain treatments and diagnostics, hospital flow, and the availability of adequate facilities to examine and treat patients did not differ between the groups. On the other hand, corporate practitioners reported more tangible benefits, such as insurance and continuing education. However, they also reported more pressure to generate revenue and seeing more clients per shift. While definitive conclusions cannot be drawn as to why, particularly for the 46% of practitioners who would prefer private practice currently work in corporate practice despite their preferences, the financial benefits could be a balancing factor for some of the increased job demands. In contrast, private practitioners reported higher satisfaction in their personal relationships with management, hospital culture, autonomy, and mentorship, which could balance the decrease in financial resources seen in these roles (Kogan and Rishniw 2024).

There is certainly some individuality to the impact of any particular demand, partially due to available resources, and careful attention should be paid to finding the right balance for yourself and your current life circumstances. For instance, an overwhelming majority of relief (i.e. someone who fills in for a practice on a temporary basis) and mobile (i.e. a self-employed practice owner who does not work out of a central office) doctors reported satisfaction with work–life balance and their availability for children and other family members (Kogan and Rishniw 2024). This suggests that relief and mobile practice may be particularly attractive for people with family responsibilities, as is illustrated by Story 7.1 from a veterinarian. Their experiences show that a change in life

STORY 7.1 SCHEDULE AUTONOMY FOR RELIEF VETERINARIANS

I fell into relief after contract negotiations fell through at a corporate hospital a few years ago. It ended up being for the best, as I am managing the affairs of my elderly mom who has been sick the past year. So, I need to be away from home for weeks at a time, and I also have a chronic autoimmune disease. Being able to control my schedule is a godsend. I enjoy moving around to different hospitals and working with different people. It's really reduced my stress level.

circumstances, such as a personal illness or an ill family member, can change priorities and the importance of a resource like schedule autonomy. However, these practitioners faced challenges, including the need to constantly adapt to new hospital protocols, limited support from colleagues, and a lack of job security (Kogan and Rishniw 2024). This lack of consistency and support might make these roles a poor fit for new graduates who need mentorship. For a practitioner to feel satisfied with their role as a relief or mobile doctor, schedule flexibility needs to be a strong enough benefit to outweigh concerns about job security and consistency. As reported by some mobile and relief doctors, demands in other, more traditional associate roles, such as rigid schedules or coworker conflict, were felt to be more taxing than issues of job security and adapting to new protocols. There is no "one size fits all" job that is perfect for every veterinary professional. However, there are certainly overall themes that can be either harmful or protective of well-being. In the remainder of the chapter, we explore elements of culture that can be burdensome or beneficial to employee well-being.

LEADERSHIP

Simon Sinek, acclaimed author, stated, "[Workplace] culture matters. How management chooses to treat its people impacts everything for better or for worse." Certainly, this idea is true in veterinary medicine. A survey of a corporate practice in Canada found that leadership quality significantly influenced employees' commitment to their workplace (Janke et al. 2023). So, what does a good leader look like? The study noted three leadership attributes linked to positive employee engagement: the ability to prioritize job satisfaction, effective work planning, and adept conflict resolution (Janke et al. 2023). Conflict and its resolution are covered in Chapter 6. In this section, we explore leadership styles as well as key elements of work planning and their impact on well-being.

LEADERSHIP PRIORITIES AND JOB SATISFACTION

Practice management involves balancing a variety of often competing interests. The needs of sick animals frequently outpace the availability of appointments. Clients must feel taken care of. The practice must stay profitable to survive. Shifts must be filled. Bills must be paid. It's easy to see where even a well-intentioned leader might lose sight of their team's well-being. At the end of the day, it's a matter of priorities and core values. When faced with two competing demands, what choice does a leader make? Let's look at the following example of a leader's reaction to competing demands.

> *I got injured doing a laceration repair on my lunch break on a Sunday. I was already super stressed because it was the pandemic, and we were fully booked in appointments and seeing walk-ins. Anyway, the dog bit my dominant hand, and I could not function. The hand surgeon I was referred to told me I could not safely work until it healed. Still, every 48 hours, I got a text from my manager asking me to move up rechecks. I was told I was stressing out staff by making them reschedule things due to my injury. It is hard enough being injured. I really didn't need someone else trying to lay blame and guilt on me for an incident I had no control over. I didn't want to be hurt, but I was. If anyone was at fault, it was the manager and the clinic's policies. We were pushed to go so fast, never take breaks, never turn down a walk-in, and I got hurt. I got zero support, and it made me so angry. Even when I did come back, I still couldn't handle a large dog or do certain procedures. They refused to even make that accommodation in my schedule. I quit three weeks later.*

In our most empathetic moment, we can understand that this situation has placed stressors on management. If the doctor does not come in, injured and sick pets will experience delayed care. Clients will be inconvenienced. The practice will lose revenue, and staff hours (and paychecks) could be negatively affected. These are all practical considerations for the business. However, placing these concerns above an employee's physical safety and emotional well-being contributes to a toxic work environment. Pressuring this doctor to come in and blaming them for an accident does not put this doctor's well-being first. While that doctor may even understand and agree with the competing demands, this leader has signaled their priorities lie with the needs of the clinic first. In this case, this leadership behavior caused the clinic to permanently lose a doctor, and those short-term concerns became long-term problems as the clinic was forced to recruit another doctor.

In the late 1970s, the concept of positive leadership, or leadership that focuses on influencing positive emotions of team members, began to gain traction (Hoch et al., 2018). Burns (1978) described this as transformational vs transactional leadership. While transactional leadership focuses on short-term goals, financial rewards, and self-interest, transformational leadership focuses on encouraging followers' personal development and achievement through communication and the instillation of trust and pride in the organization. There is a large body of literature supporting transformational leadership in terms of leader effectiveness, job satisfaction, engagement, and employee retention (Hock 2017). In the above example with the injured doctor, we saw a transactional approach – focused on the short-term issue of delayed appointments – and saw how it led to a poor outcome for everyone involved.

Under the positive leadership umbrella, other models, including ethical, authentic, and servant, have also been shown to have a positive impact on workplace performance and culture (Hoch et al. 2018). Central to all of these models are interactions between leadership and their teams that focus on building a positive work culture first and financial success second. In his 1977 book, Rober Greenleaf describes the concept of servant leadership:

> *... make sure that other people's highest priority needs are being served. The best test is: do those served grow as persons; do they, while being served, become healthier, wiser, freer, more autonomous, more likely themselves to become servants?*
>
> (Greenleaf 1977)

By prioritizing employee needs, positive leaders set the stage for workplace satisfaction. Story 7.2 is an example of positive leadership and its power to make a new employee feel valued and cared for on their first day.

Interestingly, Janke (2023) also found a potential downside to effective leaders with a high commitment to the workplace, and that is work–life conflict. All employees, including leaders, who are highly vested in their workplaces may lose sight of the important balance between one's personal and professional selves. Therefore, a leader who is truly committed to well-being must ensure that the demands of the workplace do not place undue toll on team members' free time (including their own). A big part of achieving that balance is effective work planning.

STORY 7.2 SERVANT LEADERSHIP

It was my first day at a new job as a medical director. The CEO was there to greet me. She realized the new office chair had not been assembled yet and immediately got on the floor to put it together and make sure it was ready. She was tightening the screws herself when I arrived and apologized that she was not ready for me. That level of "I will make it happen and you deserve to be cared for" was awesome.

EFFECTIVE WORK PLANNING

Work planning can take many forms. Once job roles and expectations are clearly set, it's up to the management to orchestrate the symphony of a practice's workflow. From caseload to hours and staffing, management plays a key role in setting the parameters within which their team will work. The delicate balance between the needs of the patients and the needs of the team can be difficult to achieve. When it goes wrong, the team feels overloaded and may experience work–life conflict, both of which have negative impacts on well-being. In fact, in a survey of 11,627 US veterinarians, overwork and long hours were the most frequently cited stressors facing the profession (Nett et al. 2015). This is an area where practice management has a key role.

However, the formula for success is not as simple as working fewer hours and, as a result, experiencing less work overload. In fact, in an assessment of the impact that the number of hours worked has on well-being, Volk found that working *fewer* hours than desired had more than twice the negative impact on well-being than working too many hours (Volk et al. 2020). Once again, there is an aspect of personal balance that comes into play. Other factors contribute to the balance as well, such as schedule predictability, the type of hours worked, and staffing levels. In Chapter 9, we will address the impact of the workplace on individual-level factors like work–life balance and burnout. In this chapter, we are focused on the system-level factors that can be modified to positively impact well-being.

Consistency and Predictability

Schedule inconsistency has been associated with psychological distress, sleep disturbance, and lower happiness (Schneider and Harknett 2019). The most obvious impact of an unpredictable schedule is financial insecurity. When an hourly or production-based employee cannot predict when and how many hours they will work, it becomes difficult to create a budget. However, financial insecurity is not the only reason schedule inconsistency reduces job satisfaction and well-being. In one study, hourly workers stated they would be willing to take a 20% pay cut in order to have schedule changes made at least a week in advance (Mas and Pallais 2017). So, if not purely a financial problem, why does an unstable schedule impact well-being?

Work–life conflict is an important consideration. If you cannot predict your hours, it's difficult to schedule the rest of your life. This can be a particular pain point for workers with small children, as arranging childcare is severely impacted by irregular scheduling. In fact, in a 2019 survey, work–life interference was shown to have greater impacts on psychological distress and sleep than financial insecurity (Schneider and Harknett 2019). Given these results, it seems reasonable to focus attention on creating predictable schedules for employees. If a set schedule is not possible, it can help to release the schedule well in advance to maximize employees' abilities to schedule outside responsibilities and activities around work.

Type of Hours Worked

The type of hours worked can also affect employees' well-being. For instance, night shifts and on-call work are associated with poor well-being, work–life conflict, depression, and interrupted sleep (Karhula et al. 2020; Kogan et al. 2020). Additionally, night shift work has measurable negative impacts on physical health, including an increase in general, cardiovascular, and cancer mortality (Su et al. 2021). Among veterinarians specifically, working evening, weekend, and holiday hours is associated with reduced well-being (Volk et al. 2020). On-call hours, even if the individual is not called in to work, can also have negative effects. Extended availability has been related to problems with recovery, job satisfaction, poorer well-being, and work–life interference in the general population and in veterinary medicine specifically (Kogan 2021; Steffey et al. 2023; Mas and Pallais 2017).

Given the negative impacts of night shifts or on-call work on well-being and physical health, the simplest answer would be for veterinary professionals not to engage in this type of work. However, we work in a field where emergencies happen, and there would be dire consequences if everyone closed their doors at 5 p.m. Certainly, in urban centers there has been a shift from in-house emergency care to referral emergency care, which can relieve the burden on the rest of the professional community. Yet, this solution is not yet practical in all settings. Rural markets may not be large enough to sustain an independent emergency hospital, and travel distances to the closest emergency center may be impractical for medical emergencies. Similarly, given the difficulty of transport and other considerations, referral to emergency centers is often not practical in equine and large animal work. So how is the veterinary professional to balance their personal well-being with the reality that veterinary healthcare availability does not conform to standard nine to five hours?

Literature from the human healthcare field offers one solution in the form of work time autonomy. Schedule autonomy, or the control an employee has over their schedule, has been shown to reduce work–life interference as well as lower sleep difficulties and fatigue in human healthcare professionals working night shifts (Karhula et al. 2020). Schedule autonomy has also been found to significantly reduce burnout in veterinary technicians and play a key role in job satisfaction among relief and mobile veterinarians (Kogan 2020, 2024).

However, it's important to acknowledge that complete schedule autonomy may be challenging to achieve in a clinic setting. It may not be feasible, for example, for employees to choose when their shift begins or ends. Yet, schedule autonomy is not an all-or-nothing proposition. Even if the time of the shift cannot be changed, the ability to take time off when desired could help mitigate the negative impact of rigid shift lengths. Other examples include the ability to decline a case that would extend work hours past the scheduled shift or the ability to take a break during the shift. Management should endeavor to enhance schedule autonomy in whatever ways are possible. We discuss other forms of autonomy as an important predictor of well-being later in this chapter.

Work Overload

Work overload, often recognized by a lack of downtime, is also frequently listed as a source of stress in veterinary settings (Ashton-James and McNeilage 2022). For example, a majority of polled vets reported neither being able to routinely take a lunch break nor having time allocated in their day to catch up on necessary administrative tasks like paperwork (Ashton-James and McNeilage 2022; Hilton et al. 2023). Additionally, this study found that approximately 25% of polled veterinarians did not think they could take a holiday in the next year or take sick leave on short notice (Hilton et al. 2023). This paints a picture of a workload that exceeds available resources, forcing veterinary teams to sacrifice reasonable breaks and time to keep up with paperwork/callbacks. Unsurprisingly, this type of overload correlates with depression, anxiety, stress, and a lack of job appreciation. As was discussed with schedule concerns, control over the daily structure has been found to be a significant moderator of distress (Hilton et al. 2023).

Staffing

Another common topic when discussing work overload is staffing; 71% of polled team members in a recent study reported feeling staff shortages are a critical challenge in the field (Volk et al. 2024). Concern for widespread shortages in small animal medicine became commonplace during the COVID-19 pandemic, joining long-standing shortage concerns in large animal, government, and specialty medicine (Prince et al. 2006; Zhang 2022). In 2024, a study based on the 10-year projections of occupational growth and turnover from the US Bureau of Labor Statistics found that the projected veterinary graduates (~53,000) will meet only about 76% of the US need for veterinarians (Gitter and LaFayette 2024).

Insufficient staffing has been repeatedly identified as a risk factor in well-being (Connolly et al. 2022; Hayes et al. 2020; Hilton et al. 2023). Ideal staffing ratios for well-being have not been established; however, in terms of practice productivity, highly efficient practices have, on average, 3.2 veterinarians and 5.7 clinical team members (credentialed technicians and assistants). Additionally, practices with a higher ratio of credentialed technicians vs assistants showed greater efficiency (Ouedraogo et al. 2023). Given the data on the importance of technicians in practice productivity, it is unfortunate that 60% of technicians feel underutilized at their jobs (NAVTA

2022a). Skills utilization has been shown to be protective against burnout, so better staffing and better utilization of team members provide a win-win for practice productivity and workplace well-being (Kogan et al. 2020).

PRACTICE OWNER WELL-BEING

From the above sections, we can see that much of the responsibility falls on practice leadership. Although it has become increasingly uncommon for veterinary practices to be owned by veterinarians (Teller 2023), we want to devote some consideration to practice ownership, which introduces a distinct constellation of stressors beyond those experienced by associates. Owners have additional financial responsibilities for profitability, payroll, and capital investment, while navigating client price sensitivity and rising operational costs (Vande Griek et al. 2018; AVMA 2025). Administrative demands, such as human resources, legal compliance, and marketing, consume significant time and often encroach on clinical duties (Campbell et al. 2023). Workforce shortages heighten pressure to recruit and retain skilled staff, and owners must mediate interpersonal conflicts and maintain team morale (AVMA 2025), on top of their clinical duties.

Practice owners frequently describe feeling overextended by the dual demands of clinical care and business management, citing responsibility for profitability, bookkeeping, staffing, and regulatory compliance as major sources of stress, particularly given limited formal preparation in business management during veterinary training (Campbell et al. 2023; AVMA 2025). Fewer than half of owners report feeling adequately prepared for business or leadership responsibilities by their veterinary education, underscoring the gap between clinical training and the realities of ownership (AVMA 2025).

So how do these stressors impact well-being? Surprisingly, practice owners tend to do better than associates in terms of well-being. In a large, matched-cohort study of over 2,600 US veterinarians, practice owners scored better in compassion satisfaction, with only 42.7% of owners reporting low compassion satisfaction compared to 53.8% of associates. There was a trend, although not significant, toward lower burnout among practice owners (mean 26.1 vs 26.9), despite no difference in secondary traumatic stress scores (Ouedraogo et al. 2022). Additional studies have shown that associates are approximately twice as likely to report lower job satisfaction and higher burnout compared with practice owners (Steffey et al. 2023).

These data suggest that despite being exposed to a similar, if not greater, stressors, practice owners are more resistant to that stress than associates. There are no definitive data as to why this is. It may be that practice ownership attracts particularly resilient individuals, but broader studies on workplace well-being suggest that autonomy plays a role in this context (Tummers and Bakker 2021). The practice owner in Story 7.3 shares the reasons practice

STORY 7.3 THE JOYS OF PRACTICE OWNERSHIP

The worst day as an owner is still better than the best day as an associate for me. I love bonding with clients and having the autonomy to do best for my patients, even when it isn't a good financial decision. One of my favorite clients was a woman in her 90s who would yell at me if I gave her discounts, so I would manually adjust all her prices down so I could charge her less without her knowing. She left me her cat in her will. I love mentoring, and over two dozen of my previous employees are now in vet school or practicing vets (most of them specialists). My employees are family to me. I honestly love and care about them. I love having the power to tell mean clients that they can't come back so I can focus my attention on the nice ones. Sometimes I think about how most people work in an office all day with exactly zero animals in it, and I get to see a new very good boy or very good girl every 30 minutes, and I realize I am so freakin lucky!

ownership was a good choice for them, including autonomy over things like firing clients and adjusting prices.

AUTONOMY AND SKILL UTILIZATION

In the JD-R model, one of the resources most commonly referenced is autonomy. Autonomy, or the ability to decide how to perform your own job, has been linked to reduced job stress and improved employee well-being and engagement broadly, and both veterinarians and support team members specifically (Ashton-James and McNeilage 2022; Hilton et al. 2023; Kogan et al. 2020; Rohlf 2022; Tummers and Bakker 2021). This is in contrast to job authority, or having control over others' work, which can detrimentally impact well-being (Davis 2019).

Autonomy in veterinary practice can take many forms. Story 7.4 demonstrates what can happen when autonomy is removed. Clearly, what seems to have been a small decision, to not allow veterinarians to use their preferred macros, had a far-reaching impact. Opportunities to enhance autonomy are plentiful in daily practice (see Table 7.1), and leaders are encouraged to allow for autonomy whenever practical.

In addition to deciding how and when the work is accomplished, veterinary teams also want to feel like their skills are being utilized appropriately (Kogan et al. 2020; Mastenbroek et al. 2014). This is particularly important to veterinary technicians and assistants (Wallace 2019). The ability to use one's skills and knowledge is key to mitigating burnout and to making work meaningful (Cake et al. 2015). Recognition for individuals' efforts and contributions to the shared goal of providing the best animal care is one strategy that leaders can use to support technicians and make them feel a valued part of the animal health care team (Kogan 2020).

STORY 7.4 LOSS OF AUTONOMY

We had been bought by a corporation, and they were having us change to a new computer system, which was frustrating enough. However, even through all the normal growing pains of learning a new piece of software, the number one most frustrating thing is that they would not allow doctors to add any macros or documents to the system. I have literally a decade of handouts I've written, macros that make writing my records easier, and they were all gone in a split second. The specialists at the practice were furious, as we had poured a tremendous amount of effort into our records and client handouts. Most of us have written small novels on patient diseases and care, and in a moment, they all got flushed. In that small act, they not only made every single part of my day harder, but they told me loud and clear that I wasn't allowed to do things my way even in the smallest things. It was an early signal that I wasn't important to them as an individual. I was just a cog in their machine. I left that practice within a year.

Table 7.1 Opportunities for autonomy in practice.

Examples of autonomy in practice include the ability to:
• Fire a client
• Turn down a case
• Take a break when desired
• Take PTO when desired
• Control over diagnostic and treatment choices to align with your professional judgment
• Access and utilize resources that you find helpful (e.g. using a phone app instead of a textbook)

CULTURE OF COMMUNICATION

A team that communicates effectively and works well together is consistently listed as a source of workplace well-being (Ashton-James and McNeilage 2022; McKee et al. 2021). In a survey of veterinary nurses in the UK, good communication was found to be a key contributor to positive well-being (Vivian et al. 2022). In a large survey of veterinarians, 98% of those polled said that communication skills were equal to or more important than clinical knowledge (McDermott et al. 2015). So what does good communication look like within the workplace? Key elements include shared values and goals, role clarity, diagonal communication, and conflict resolution. Conflict resolution is covered in Chapter 6.

SHARED VALUES AND GOALS

Core values encapsulate the fundamental beliefs and philosophies that govern how individuals within the organization interact and make decisions. Complete alignment of values is not necessary for a harmonious workplace. Employees and organizations can still find alignment in achieving a shared goal, even if they approach it from different value-based frameworks (Guillemin and Nicholas 2022).

The first step to shared goals is clearly communicating both the goal and the values at play. See Figure 7.2. for examples of some common workplace values in veterinary medicine. All of these values have positive aspects, but they can conflict with one another. A practice that values efficiency over, say, customer service would likely favor a higher caseload rather than more contact time with clients. There can also be a values conflict within the team. In Story 7.5, a practice owner discusses the conflict that arose with their lead technician over conflicting values and how they resolved it through compromise and communication – particularly by centering the resolution on their shared value of staff happiness, which led to a satisfying outcome for all involved.

ROLE CLARITY

People cannot thrive in their roles without knowing precisely what those roles entail. Unfortunately, in veterinary work environments, this clarity is not always present, often causing significant distress (Nett 2015; Perry 2020). For example, title protection and clear practice acts are not universally available to credentialed technicians in the United States. According to NAVTA's review of

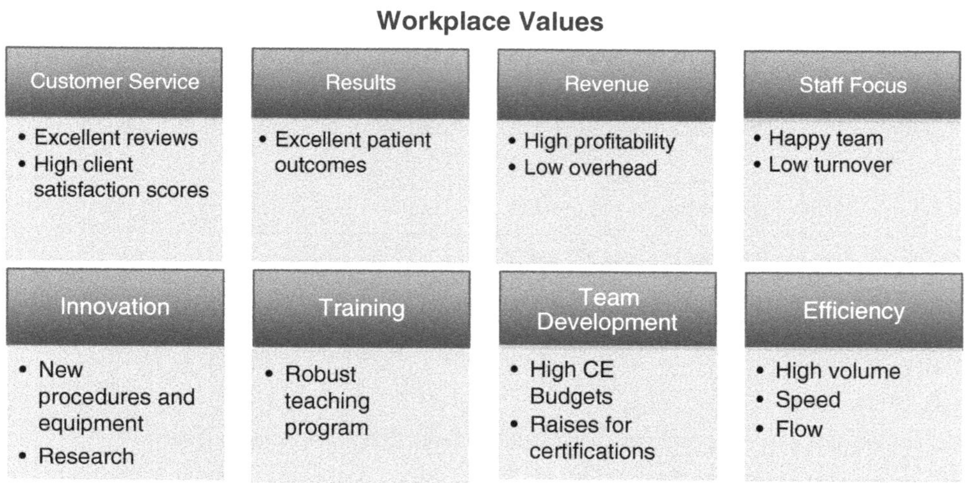

FIGURE 7.2 Examples of common workplace-oriented values, as well as examples of how those values may show up in practice.

STORY 7.5 VALUES CONFLICT

As a practice owner, I value my team over everything else. My business partners and I started the practice so we could work with people I like and treat them well. However, if I'm being honest, I also really like efficiency, and if we want to keep the practice running, we have to think about revenue. Early on, I butted heads with my lead technician/business partner over a few issues. He's definitely someone who always wants to do the newest thing. He wants us to try the newest drug, learn the latest procedures, and he genuinely enjoys teaching. I very much want him to be happy, but new techniques aren't always better than established ones. New drugs are often more expensive and can have unforeseen complications. And while theoretically I am a big fan of having a well-trained team, it makes me want to pull my hair out when I see he's having the brand-new assistant place the catheter, when one of the other techs could do it in a third of the time.

So, we talked it over and reached some agreements. Before we try a new drug or procedure, he has to bring me evidence as to why it's an improvement over what we already do. He also has to do a price analysis to prove that it's at least as profitable as the current one. In return, I've had to chill out about him taking time to train. I know it's good for us in the long haul, so I just take some deep breaths and let him do it. We both want everyone to enjoy working here. That means he gets to do some training, which the team loves, and I get a happy team that, in the long run, is at the top of its game.

state practice acts, 31 states and jurisdictions have no title protection for veterinary technicians, 10 have limited title protection, and only 11 provide general protection restricting the use of "veterinary technician" to credentialed individuals (NAVTA 2022b). A recent NAVTA report found that 54% of respondents indicated feeling that credentialed and uncredentialed veterinary techs are trained to perform the same job duties, which can lead to resentment (Friesen 2023).

Role clarity can take many forms. A position within a practice should have a clearly defined job description. This description should outline both desirable skills and duties. Roles, duties, and goals can be further clarified in employee review sessions. Role clarity can also be achieved more casually. For example, before each morning's appointments, a hospital team could review which staff members will run the appointments and which will perform procedures. In addition, hospitals can help employees differentiate credentialed techs from assistants through visual cues such as name tags and differently colored scrubs, ensuring everyone can work within their level of knowledge and training. Currently, five states (California, Indiana, Georgia, New York, and Oklahoma) require visual identification cues for role clarity, such as name tags with titles and license numbers clearly displayed.

DIAGONAL COMMUNICATION

Workplace communication occurs in three forms: vertical, lateral, and diagonal. Vertical communication happens between different organizational levels (e.g. manager and employee), lateral communication occurs among peers (e.g. receiving tech and intensive care unit [ICU] tech), and diagonal communication crosses departments or roles (e.g. ICU technician to surgeon). Diagonal communication bypasses formal hierarchies and fosters open, respectful dialogue, but it can be challenging to establish in medicine's hierarchical culture.

Even when they do not have a specific management role, doctors guide patient care, writing orders for technicians and assistants to carry out. This structure, unfortunately, reinforces a dynamic of deference to authority that can impact workplace culture and communication. This may not only negatively affect employees' emotional well-being, but also patient care. Reports suggest that upwards of 70% of all medical errors are communication-related, with nearly a quarter caused by a failure of someone lower in the hierarchy to speak up (Peadon 2020).

When faced with this statistic, many in leadership roles can be in denial about their contributions to this problem, believing they are approachable. In fact, in a survey of surgery residents and their mentors, mentors universally agreed that they encourage residents to speak up if they have questions about medical decision-making. Unfortunately, only 55% of their residents agreed (Belyansky et al. 2011). Even more troubling is that 53% of residents recalled a time when they felt unable to voice a concern and that this resulted in an adverse event. These statistics suggest the need for an active focus on flattening the hierarchies within veterinary practices (vertical communication) and on encouraging diagonal communication (Belyansky et al. 2011).

Within the veterinary team, those at the bottom of the organizational tree, customer service representatives and unlicensed assistants, have the lowest well-being scores (Volk et al., 2024b). While the reasons for this are certainly multifactorial, the responsibility for flattening this hierarchy lies primarily with those at the top. It starts with building familiarity and relationships. Comfort in speaking up is shaped not only by organizational culture but also by interpersonal dynamics and personality-linked factors such as confidence, assertiveness, and perceived efficacy. Individuals who feel comfortable and supported by senior colleagues are significantly more likely to voice concerns (Peadon et al. 2020). Following through on this theme, senior team members must show a willingness to take feedback and, more importantly, to act on it or address their team's needs. It is also important for leaders to be cognizant of the power dynamics at play and the level of risk that their team members may feel when speaking up.

Once we have flattened the hierarchy in our work environments, we open the door to better communication. Effective communication fosters a sense of value and respect and cohesion within the team, which in turn is protective for well-being in both veterinarians and technicians (Ashton-James 2022, Kogan et al. 2020, Kogan and Rishniw 2024; Vivian 2022). Elements of communication that can help foster the culture we want in the workplace include helping people feel safe, both physically and psychologically, so they feel free to speak without fear of retribution or negative judgment. Additionally, it is important to recognize and praise all team members, showing appreciation and gratitude for their contributions and ideas (Hicks and Stiles, 2021).

FEEDBACK

Part of being a functional team is feedback. A growth-oriented culture encourages people at all levels to exchange constructive feedback, yet this is not always valued. In a study of veterinary specialty residents, trainees highly valued two-way feedback, while their mentors did not (Perry 2020), underscoring the need for buy-in from leadership.

Effective feedback depends on both content and delivery. Team members must be able to receive as well as give feedback (Scott 2017), and communication should be predominantly positive. In business teams, the most successful groups offered about six positive comments for every negative, compared with three positive comments to one negative comment in the least successful teams (Losada and Heaphy 2004). In Story 7.6, a technician discusses the importance of positive feedback to her overall happiness at a practice.

STORY 7.6 POSITIVE FEEDBACK

My new ICU supervisor personally thanked me for showing a couple coworkers through a central line placement. Added in "it was really nice to see how much happier you are when teaching, you can tell it's something you enjoy." I would have left this practice otherwise; it was a relief to have a supportive supervisor who listened.

Start feedback from inquiry: state an observation, then ask for perspective – "I noticed you struggled with that procedure; what made today hard?" High-performing teams ask as many questions as they give statements of their opinion, while low performers state opinions 20 times per question (Losada and Heaphy 2004). Asking invites reflection and context (Peadon 2020) – perhaps in the above example the difficulty with the procedure came from a migraine, not lack of skill.

Feedback should aim for growth rather than criticism (Oxtoby and Mossop 2019). Because veterinary professionals often self-punish for mistakes (Kogan et al. 2018), a nonretaliatory tone matters. Reframing "What did you do?" to "What happened today?" removes blame and fosters problem-solving. Ideally, the person receiving feedback guides the improvement plan, aligning it with their values and habits.

MENTORSHIP

Another key form of communication is around mentorship. Mentorship benefits veterinary professionals at all stages but is especially critical early in their careers. Well-being studies consistently show higher stress in younger veterinarians (Volk et al. 2020), and about 44% of new graduates leave their first job within a year, often citing inadequate mentorship (Gates et al. 2020). This highlights the need for structured support.

Traditionally, mentorship pairs a senior team member with a junior colleague to guide professional growth. Early conversations should clarify expectations, including how much supervision is desired, comfort with independence or on-call duty, and the availability of backup, since preferences vary widely.

Setting milestones improves clarity. In a residency survey, both residents and supervisors reported a lack of defined benchmarks and wanted structured skill lists (Perry 2020). Even outside residencies, many graduates and mentors value technical skills checklists, while soft skills such as communication or financial management are often overlooked despite being common stressors (Routly et al. 2002; Veterinary Schools and Royal College of Veterinary Surgeons 2020). Mentorship focused on these areas has been shown to reduce stress and improve well-being (Reinhard 2021).

Beyond traditional one-to-one arrangements, more informal mentorship models can enrich learning and build community. Peer-to-peer mentorship allows colleagues to share skills directly, such as a technician teaching another to use new equipment. Group mentorship leverages the strengths of multiple team members, enabling each person to contribute their expertise. This creates a more well-rounded experience and reduces reliance on a single mentor. When all team members are encouraged to teach and learn from each other, mentorship becomes a shared responsibility that strengthens collaboration, supports professional identity, and fosters a culture where growth and feedback are part of everyday practice.

CONCLUSION

Workplace culture exerts a powerful influence on both team functioning and individual well-being. Environments that emphasize psychological safety, equitable communication, and shared growth enable team members to contribute more effectively and experience greater engagement (Ashton-James 2022, Kogan et al. 2020, Kogan and Rishniw 2024; Vivian 2022). Effective work planning – through clear expectations, appropriate workload, autonomy, and opportunities for skill development – further strengthens engagement and buffers against stress (Mastenbroek et al. 2014; Volk et al. 2024). Addressing hierarchical barriers and fostering open dialogue enhances trust and reduces communication-related errors (Peadon 2020; Belyansky et al. 2011). By intentionally aligning organizational culture with evidence-based principles of communication, feedback, and structured planning, veterinary teams can build environments that support well-being, sustain motivation, and improve the quality of patient care.

REFERENCES

Andela, M. (2020). Burnout, somatic complaints, and suicidal ideations among veterinarians: development and validation of the Veterinarians Stressors Inventory. *Journal of Veterinary Behavior* 37: 48–55.

Ashton-James, C.E. and McNeilage, A.G. (2022). A mixed methods investigation of stress and wellbeing factors contributing to burnout and job satisfaction in a specialist small animal hospital. *Frontiers in Veterinary Science* 9: 942778.

AVMA (2025). *Economic State of the Veterinary Profession 2025*. Schaumburg, IL: American Veterinary Medical Association.

Bakker, A.B., Demerouti, E., and Sanz-Vergel, A. (2023). Job demands–resources theory: ten years later. *Annual Review of Organizational Psychology and Organizational Behavior* 10: 25–53.

Behfar, K.J., Peterson, R.S., Mannix, E.A., and Trochim, W.M. (2008). The critical role of conflict resolution in teams: a close look at the links between conflict type, conflict management strategies, and team outcomes. *Journal of Applied Psychology* 93 (1): 170.

Belyansky, I., Martin, T.R., Prabhu, A.S. et al. (2011). Poor resident-attending intraoperative communication may compromise patient safety. *Journal of Surgical Research* 171 (2): 386–394.

Berrada, M., Ndiaye, Y., Raboisson, D., and Lhermie, G. (2022). Spatial evaluation of animal health care accessibility and veterinary shortage in France. *Scientific Reports* 12 (1): 13022.

Burns, J.M. (1978). *Leadership*. New York: Harper & Row.

Cake, M.A., Bell, M.A., Bickley, N., and Bartram, D.J. (2015). The life of meaning: a model of the positive contributions to well-being from veterinary work. *Journal of Veterinary Medical Education* 42 (3): 184–193.

Campbell, J., Kogan, L., and Schoenfeld-Tacher, R. (2023). Veterinarians' experiences of stress and mental health: a qualitative study. *Frontiers in Veterinary Science* 10: 1064932.

Christian, K. (2020). *Finding Confidence in Conflict: How to Negotiate Anything and Live Your Best Life*. Columbus, OH: American Negotiation Institute LLC.

Connolly, C.E., Norris, K., Martin, A. et al. (2022). A taxonomy of occupational and organisational stressors and protectors of mental health reported by veterinary professionals in Australasia. *Australian Veterinary Journal* 100 (8): 367–376.

Dantas, L.A. and Cunha, A. (2020). An integrative debate on learning styles and the learning process. *Social Sciences & Humanities Open* 2 (1): 100017.

Davis, A.L. (2019). Job Control in Professional Practice: A Study on the Implications for Well-Being. Master's thesis. University of Calgary, Calgary.

Dawson, B.F. and Thompson, N.J. (2017). The effect of personality on occupational stress in veterinary surgeons. *Journal of Veterinary Medical Education* 44 (1): 72–83.

Dicks, M.R. (2013). A short history of veterinary workforce analyses. *Journal of the American Veterinary Medical Association* 242 (8): 1051–1060.

Doherty, C. (2020). The demand for associate veterinarians: surveying the "shortage". *The Canadian Veterinary Journal* 61 (1): 85.

Fletcher, K., 2023. Relation of a career ladder professional development approach to employee engagement: a qualitative within-site case study of veterinary technical staff within a veterinary teaching hospital.

Friesen, M., 2023. Navta survey reveals veterinary technician pay and education have increased, but burnout, debt are still issues. *NAVTA, February, 14.*

Gates, M.C., McLachlan, I., Butler, S., and Weston, J.F. (2020). Experiences of recent veterinary graduates in their first employment position and their preferences for new graduate support programmes. *New Zealand Veterinary Journal* 68 (4): 214–224.

Gitter, R.J. and LaFayette, B. (2024). *Demand for and Supply of Veterinarians in the U.S. to 2032*. Washington, DC: American Association of Veterinary Medical Colleges (AAVMC).

Greenleaf, R.K., 1977. Servant leadership: A journey into the nature of legitimate power and greatness. New York: Paulist.

Groysberg, B., Lee, J., Price, J., and Cheng, J. (2018). The leader's guide to corporate culture. *Harvard Business Review* 96 (1): 44–52.

Guillemin, M. and Nicholas, R. (2022). Core values at work—essential elements of a healthy workplace. *International Journal of Environmental Research and Public Health 19* (19): 12505.

Hagen, J.R., Weller, R., Mair, T.S., and Kinnison, T. (2020). Investigation of factors affecting recruitment and retention in the UK veterinary profession. *Veterinary Record* 187 (9): 354–354.

Hayes, G.M., LaLonde-Paul, D.F., Perret, J.L. et al. (2020). Investigation of burnout syndrome and job-related risk factors in veterinary technicians in specialty teaching hospitals: a multicenter cross-sectional study. *Journal of Veterinary Emergency and Critical Care* 30 (1): 18–27.

Hicks M. and Stiles E. or Canadian Veterinary Medical Association (2021) '2020 Annual Report of the Canadian Veterinary Medical Association', The Canadian Veterinary Journal, 62(7), pp. 687–711.

Hilton, K.R., Burke, K.J., and Signal, T. (2023). Mental health in the veterinary profession: an individual or organisational focus? *Australian Veterinary Journal* 101 (1–2): 41–48.

Hoch, J.E., Bommer, W.H., Dulebohn, J.H., and Wu, D. (2018). Do ethical, authentic, and servant leadership explain variance above and beyond transformational leadership? *A meta-analysis. Journal of management* 44 (2): 501–529.

Hurley, J. and Hutchinson, M. (2020). Hierarchy and medical error: speaking up when witnessing an error. *Safety Science* 125: 104648.

Janke, N., Gohar, B., Blokland, K., and Coe, J.B. (2023). Workplace psychosocial factors are associated with veterinary employees' organizational commitment to their current veterinary hospital. *Journal of the American Veterinary Medical Association* 1 (aop): 1–10.

Karhula, K., Turunen, J., Hakola, T. et al. (2020). The effects of using participatory working time scheduling software on working hour characteristics and wellbeing: a quasi-experimental study of irregular shift work. *International Journal of Nursing Studies* 112: 103696.

Kimber, S. and Gardner, D. (2016). Relationships between workplace wellbeing, job demands and resources in a sample of veterinary nurses in New Zealand. *New Zealand Veterinary Journal* 64 (4): 224–229.

Kogan, L., Schoenfeld-Tacher, R., Carney, P. et al. (2021). On-call duties: the perceived impact on veterinarians' job satisfaction, well-being and personal relationships. *Frontiers in veterinary science* 8: 740852.

Kogan, L.R., Booth, M., and Rishniw, M. (2022). Factors that impact recruitment and retention of veterinarians in emergency practice. *Journal of the American Veterinary Medical Association* 260 (15): 1986–1992.

Kogan, L.R. and Rishniw, M. (2024). Relief and mobile veterinary careers may offer a path towards improved quality of life. *Journal of the American Veterinary Medical Association* 262 (2): 209–215.

Kogan, L.R. and Rishniw, M. (2024). Career transition plans of veterinarians in clinical practice. *Frontiers in Veterinary Science* 11: 1433891.

Kogan, L.R., Rishniw, M., Hellyer, P.W., and Schoenfeld-Tacher, R.M. (2018). Veterinarians' experiences with near misses and adverse events. *Journal of the American Veterinary Medical Association* 252 (5): 586–595.

Kogan, L.R., Wallace, J.E., Schoenfeld-Tacher, R. et al. (2020). Veterinary technicians and occupational burnout. *Frontiers in Veterinary Science* 7: 328.

Losada, M. and Heaphy, E. (2004). The role of positivity and connectivity in the performance of business teams: A nonlinear dynamics model. *American behavioral scientist* 47 (6): 740–765.

Mas, A. and Pallais, A. (2017). Valuing alternative work arrangements. *The American Economic Review* 107 (12): 3722–3759.

Mastenbroek, N.J.J.M., Jaarsma, A.D.C., Demerouti, E. et al. (2014). Burnout and engagement, and its predictors in young veterinary professionals: the influence of gender. *Veterinary Record* 174 (6): 144.

McDermott, M.P., Tischler, V.A., Cobb, M.A. et al. (2015). Veterinarian–client communication skills: current state, relevance, and opportunities for improvement. *Journal of Veterinary Medical Education* 42 (4): 305–314.

McKee, H., Gohar, B., Appleby, R. et al. (2021). High psychosocial work demands, decreased well-being, and perceived well-being needs within veterinary academia during the COVID-19 pandemic. *Frontiers in Veterinary Science* 8: 746716.

Mitchell, P., Wynia, M., Golden, R. et al. (2012). Core principles & values of effective team-based health care. *NAM Perspectives* https://doi.org/10.31478/201905A.

National Association of Veterinary Technicians in America (NAVTA) (2022a). Demographic survey results: pay & education have increased; burnout & debt are still issues. National Association of Veterinary Technicians in America. https://drive.google.com/file/d/11pmYzIouybfL55YsduRbaZ1TtMD1i2DB/view (accessed 11 February 2024).

National Association of Veterinary Technicians in America (NAVTA) (2022b). *Title Protection for "Veterinary Technician": Survey and Report Findings*, Bridgewater, NJ, 22 February.

Nett, R.J., Witte, T.K., Holzbauer, S.M. et al. (2015). Risk factors for suicide, attitudes toward mental illness, and practice-related stressors among US veterinarians. *Journal of the American Veterinary Medical Association* 247 (8): 945–955.

Ouedraogo, F.B., Bain, B., Hansen, C., and Salois, M. (2019). A census of veterinarians in the United States. *Journal of the American Veterinary Medical Association* 255 (2): 183–191.

Ouedraogo, F.B., McCullock, K., and Harris, L. (2022). Benefits of practice ownership among U.S. private veterinarians. *Journal of the American Veterinary Medical Association* 260 (15): 1790–1799.

Ouedraogo, F.B., Weinstein, P., and Lefebvre, S.L. (2023). Increased efficiency could lessen the need for more staff in companion animal practice. *Journal of the American Veterinary Medical Association* 1 (aop): 1–6.

Oxtoby, C. and Mossop, L. (2019). Blame and shame in the veterinary profession: barriers and facilitators to reporting significant events. *Veterinary Record* 184 (16): 501–501.

Peadon R, Hurley J, Hutchinson M. Hierarchy and medical error: speaking up when witnessing an error. Saf Sci 2020;125(5):104648. doi: https://doi.org/10.1016/j.ssci.2020.104648

Perry, K.L., Frendo Londgren, M., and Vinten, C. (2020). Perceptions of the feedback process: a case study of veterinary residents and supervisors. *Veterinary Record* 187 (11): 449–449.

Prince, J.B., Andrus, D.M., and Gwinner, K.P. (2006). Future demand, probable shortages, and strategies for creating a better future in food supply veterinary medicine. *Journal of the American Veterinary Medical Association* 229 (1): 57–69.

Reinhard, A.R., 2021. Stress, burnout, and well-being in new veterinary graduates: Evaluating a pilot online professional development program.

Rohlf, V.I., Scotney, R., Monaghan, H., and Bennett, P. (2022). Predictors of professional quality of life in veterinary professionals. *Journal of Veterinary Medical Education* 49 (3): 372–381.

Routly, J.E., Dobson, H., Taylor, I.R. et al. (2002). Support needs of veterinary surgeons during the first few years of practice: perceptions of recent graduates and senior partners. *Veterinary Record* 150 (6): 167–171.

Schneider, D. and Harknett, K. (2019). Consequences of routine work-schedule instability for worker health and well-being. *American Sociological Review* 84 (1): 82–114.

Scott, K. (2017). *Radical Candor: Be a Kick-Ass Boss Without Losing Your Humanity*. New York: St. Martin's Press.

Steffey, M.A., Cavanaugh, K., and Johnson, L. (2023). Veterinarian burnout demographics and organizational predictors: a cross-sectional analysis. *Frontiers in Veterinary Science* 10: 1184526.

Su, T., Li, X., Yang, Y. et al. (2021). The association between shift work and mental health: a systematic review and meta-analysis. *Sleep Medicine Reviews* 56: 101412.

Teller (2023). Straight talk about veterinary workforce issues. https://www.avma.org/news/straight-talk-about-veterinary-workforce-issues (accessed 2 March 2026)

Tummers, L.G. and Bakker, A.B. (2021). Leadership and job demands-resources theory: a systematic review. *Frontiers in Psychology* 12: 722080.

Vande Griek, O.H., Clark, M.A., Witte, T.K. et al. (2018). Development of a taxonomy of practice-related stressors experienced by veterinarians in the United States. *Journal of the American Veterinary Medical Association* 252 (2): 227–233.

Veterinary Schools Council and Royal College of Veterinary Surgeons (2020) Graduate and Employer Surveys 2019. June. Available at: https://www.vetschoolscouncil.ac.uk/wp-content/uploads/2020/06/VSC-Graduate-Employer-Surveys-2019.pdf (Accessed: 2 March 2026).

Vivian, S.R., Holt, S.L., and Williams, J. (2022). What factors influence the perceptions of job satisfaction in registered veterinary nurses currently working in veterinary practice in the United Kingdom? *Journal of Veterinary Medical Education* 49 (2): 249–259.

Volk, J.O., Schimmack, U., Strand, E.B. et al. (2024). Work-life balance is essential to reducing burnout, improving well-being. *Journal of the American Veterinary Medical Association* 262 (7): 950–957.

Volk, J.O., Schimmack, U., Strand, E.B. et al. (2024b). Merck Animal Health Veterinary Team study reveals factors associated with well-being, burnout, and mental health among nonveterinarian practice team members. *Journal of the American Veterinary Medical Association* 262 (10): 1330–1337.

Volk, J.O., Schimmack, U., Strand, E.B. et al. (2020). Executive summary of the Merck animal health veterinarian wellbeing study II. *Journal of the American Veterinary Medical Association* 256 (11): 1237–1244.

Wallace, J.E. (2019). Meaningful work and well-being: a study of the positive side of veterinary work. *Veterinary Record* 185 (18): 571.

Zhang, S. (2022). The great veterinary shortage. The Atlantic https://www.theatlantic.com/health/archive/2022/07/not-enough-veterinarians-animals/661497/ (accessed 2 November 2024).

Finances and Well-being

CHAPTER 8

Meredith Jones, DVM, CSLP®, AFC®[1]
and Carrie Jurney, DVM, DACVIM (Neurology)[2]

[1] *Allvet Financial, Richmond, VA, USA*

[2] *Not One More Vet, Inc, San Francisco, CA, USA*

INTRODUCTION

In this chapter, we discuss financial health, common financial struggles among veterinary professionals, and strategies for personal financial management.

Financial pressures and high levels of student debt are major threats to well-being and are associated with serious psychological distress among young veterinarians and veterinary team members (Volk et al. 2018, 2020, 2022, 2024). When veterinarians who said they would not recommend the veterinary profession were asked why, the two most common responses were high student debt (50%) and low compensation (45%; Volk et al. 2020).

In contrast to their impressive academic prowess, health graduate students, including veterinary school students, show poor financial literacy, scoring at most 50% correct on surveys on financial habits, credit, borrowing, and investing (Mulligan et al. 2020). Unfortunately, this lack of knowledge may also be accompanied by overconfidence in one's ability to manage finances. In a survey, 85.8% of vet students polled agreed or strongly agreed with the statement, "I am good at dealing with day-to-day financial matters." However, when asked about more involved behaviors such as checking credit scores or engaging with financial professionals, a minority of students had taken these steps (36.47% and 22.10%, respectively). One-third of these students also reported carrying credit card balances (Carr and Greenhill 2015). These statistics make the case for including financial education in veterinary schools, and, thankfully, many have added or expanded it in recent years. Some have also hired financial professionals to support their students and house officers in navigating student debt and financial planning, as well as comparing and evaluating job offers.

This chapter serves to expand on that education. Not only will there be an overview of good financial behaviors, but we will also explore links between financial health and psychological well-being. Personal finance education has been shown to be more successful if delivered at a "teachable moment," when you are able to apply your knowledge to a situation that is immediately relevant to you (Kaiser and Menkhoff 2017). For example, you may be most receptive to learning about student debt just before starting loan repayment, and you are more likely to retain information about employment benefits when you are ready to apply for a job. If you're a student, we suggest reviewing this chapter again closer to graduation and making financial education part of your continuing education.

INCOME LEVEL AND WELL-BEING

As discussed in Chapter 1, the precise connection between income and well-being has been a topic of debate in the literature. A general positive relationship between well-being and income is found across the majority of studies. However, some studies have found that the relationship dissolves above a certain level of compensation, while others find a more consistent linear relationship, and still others find a decrease in well-being above certain levels of compensation. This variation may be related to the type of well-being measured (i.e. short-term emotional well-being vs overall life satisfaction), and also a variety of other confounding factors, such as cultural norms (Jebb et al. 2018; Killingsworth 2021).

These complexities are also apparent within veterinary medicine. Satisfaction with compensation has been shown to have a positive impact on well-being among veterinary professionals (Volk et al. 2020, 2023, Kogan and Rishniw 2023, Liss et al. 2020). However, on further inspection, the relationship between compensation and well-being is, once again, complex. For instance, 59% of team members were unsatisfied with their income and financial situations, and 68% ranked compensation as critically important. However, 73% of these veterinary team members also reported mid to high levels of job satisfaction (Volk et al. 2024).

Even if income does not explain the whole of workplace well-being, it does still have a measurable impact. Economic factors also shape well-being. Lower pay contributes to financial stress, particularly among client service representatives, assistants, and entry-level technicians (Scoresby et al. 2023). While income is not the sole driver of well-being, it remains protective. Technicians earning $21 per hour or more reported higher job engagement than those earning less (Kogan et al. 2020; Liss et al. 2020), and higher income and social class levels were inversely related to psychological distress and suicidality across veterinary professionals (Scoresby et al. 2023).

FINANCIAL BASICS

According to the 2022 Merck Veterinary Wellbeing study, veterinarians who worked with a financial planner experienced lower rates of serious psychological distress and reported better overall well-being, with 60% flourishing compared to 45% without a planner (Volk et al. 2020, 2022). These veterinarians were also more likely to pay off their debts and less likely to hold credit card balances (Volk et al. 2022). Clearly, having a solid financial plan is a cornerstone of not only our financial well-being, but may also have an impact on our emotional well-being. More research is needed to establish whether financial planning leads to improved well-being, though there is clear data reflecting its impact on financial health.

A financial planner can help you evaluate the current state of your finances, prioritize your financial goals, and work collaboratively with you to develop a plan to reach your goals. Table 8.1 is based on 10 questions the Certified Financial Planner (CFP) Board recommends asking when choosing a financial advisor (CFP Board 2024). More than just nuts and bolts planning, financial counselors who use well-being theory also encourage their clients to discover how their spending aligns with their values and what they need to support their overall well-being. This "shifts the conversation away from decreasing expenses (which can be demotivating or paralyzing) to spending money where it matters (which is more motivational)" (Archuleta et al. 2019).

Table 8.1 Questions to ask your financial advisor.

What are your qualifications and credentials?
What services do you offer?
Will you have a fiduciary duty to act only in my best interest?
What is your approach to financial planning?
What types of clients do you typically work with?
Will you be the only advisor working with me?
How will I pay for your services?
How much do you typically charge?
Do others stand to gain from the financial advice you give me?
Have you ever been disciplined for any unlawful or unethical actions in your work?

Source: CFP Board / 10 Questions to Ask Your Financial Advisor/ https://www.letsmakeaplan.org/choosing-a-planner/10-questions-to-ask-your-financial-advisor/ (accessed 26 December 2025).

Unfortunately, financial planning is a resource that may be underutilized by veterinary team members, as 49% of veterinarians report having a financial advisor vs 29% and 19% of practice managers and other staff, respectively (Merck Vet Team Wellbeing 2024). However, even without a financial advisor, a basic understanding of financial matters can start us on a path to success. Although a full discussion of this topic is beyond the scope of this book, in the following section, we will give a brief overview of the foundations of financial literacy. For a more in-depth discussion, a wealth of resources on personal finance, including some tailored to the veterinary community, can be found through the AVMA (www.avma.org/resources-tools/personal-finance).

CASH FLOW PLANNING

"Budget" is a cringeworthy word for many of us, who may associate it with restriction or deprivation. The term "cash flow planning" refers to creating a plan for managing your income, expenses, and savings, which has a more positive connotation. Cash flow planning helps to form a foundation and baseline for your financial life, helping you explore how you're using your money today and how you envision using it in the future.

In her book, *All Your Worth: The Ultimate Lifetime Money Plan,* Elizabeth Warren introduced a popular budgeting strategy called the 50/30/20 rule (Warren and Tyagi 2005). With the 50/30/20 budgeting rule, you would allocate 50% of your take-home pay toward needs (housing, groceries, utilities, healthcare, and transportation), 30% toward wants (dining out, shopping, travel, entertainment, and hobbies), and 20% toward savings. Table 8.2 shows an example of two budgets using this rule. These budgets are based on the 2024 average salary of a full-time clinical veterinarian (A) or technician (B) (Kreisler et al. 2025; U.S. Bureau of Labor Statistics, 2025). Please note that factors such as location and withholdings will affect the exact posttax income. Incomes differ greatly across the veterinary team, and most support staff earn far less than veterinarians. Although they generally carry less student debt, this does not offset the financial strain created by lower wages, which can heighten stress and limit savings potential (Kogan et al. 2020; Liss et al. 2020; Scoresby et al. 2023). Recognizing these differences is important when applying budgeting strategies, as financial goals and feasible savings rates vary by compensation.

The first step in creating a plan is reviewing your income and expenses over at least three months. Since many veterinary professionals and students have variable incomes, calculating the average monthly income over at least the past few months is more accurate than using just one month. In this example, a veterinarian has a base salary of $122,500. To offset their student loan payments, they also work an average of two nights at the local emergency clinic, which pays on average $1,000 per shift. After taxes, this leaves them with a budget of $8,548. We then calculate budget targets from this number. 50% going to necessary expenses, 30% to wants, and 20% to savings.

Next, categorize and calculate your average monthly expenses by reviewing at least three months of spending. Apps like YNAB (You Need A Budget) or Monarch Money can automate this using linked accounts. Categorize your expenses in terms of necessities, wants, and savings, and then compare them to the ideal numbers you calculated based on your income. We can see in this example that the veterinarians' necessary expenses are actually more than 50% of their budget. This led the veterinarian to reduce spending on shopping and take-out food to make up for the shortfall. Finally, they have a savings plan. Currently, they are working on building an emergency fund. Once they reach their target of three months of expenses for this account, they will start saving to buy a house.

This budget leaves a net of $303 a month on average. Some expenses, like groceries and gas, are variable, which could affect this number on a month-to-month basis. If you have a surplus (positive cash flow), you have additional money that has not been designated for spending or saving, which can be allocated to financial goals such as emergency savings, consumer debt payoff, or retirement contributions. If you have a deficit (negative cash flow), you will need to borrow money, pull money from savings, and/or cut expenses to make up for the deficit.

Table 8.2 A&B Example budgets.

Example veterinary budget based on a salary of $122,500, which is the average salary after tax of a full-time clinician in 2024 according to AVMA data.							
Average posttax income							
Monthly wages		$7,028					
Other: Two emergency shifts per month		$1,520					
Total:		$8,548					
Necessary expenses							
Rent		$1,750		**Utilities**	Electricity and Gas	$0	covered in lease
Groceries		$350			Mobile	$140	
Insurance	Auto Insurance	$75			Garbage	$0	covered in lease
	Medical Insurance	$0	(covered by employer)		Internet	$75	
	Renter Insurance	$15		**Transportation**	Car payment	$415	
	Disability Insurance	$250			Gas	$150	
	Pet Insurance	$150			Car maintenance	$35	
Loans	Student Loan Payment (IBR)	$1,100					
				Total necessary expenses:		$4,505	
				Ideal budget (50% of income)		$4,274	
Wants							
Shopping: (clothing, jewelry, decor, etc.)		$200		**Travel**		$600	
Stream-ing services		$50			**Concert tickets**	$250	
Gym membership		$75			**Dining out and bars**	$450	

	Hobbies (video games, craft projects)	$165	**Take out**	$250
			Total wants	$2,040
			Ideal budget (30% of income)	$2,564
Savings				
	Emergency fund (target 30,000)	$1,200	**Saving for taxes on student loan forgiveness**	$100
	Retire-ment account	$300		
	Other investments	$100		
			Total savings	$1,700
			Ideal sudget (20% of income)	$1,710
Total expenses:	$8,245			
Net:	$303			

Example technician budget based on a salary of $45,980, which is the average salary of a full-time technician in 2024 (U.S. Bureau of Labor Statistics, 2025).

Average posttax income		
	Monthly wages	$3,750
	Other: Two nights pet sitting a month	$200
	Total:	$3,950

(*Continued*)

Table 8.2 (Continued)

Necessary expenses							
Rent		$875	(roommate pays half)	**Utilities**	Electricity and gas	$0	covered in lease
Groceries		$350			Mobile	$140	
Insurance	Auto Insurance	$75			Garbage	$0	covered in lease
	Medical Insurance	$0	(covered by employer)		Internet	$75	
	Renter Insurance	$15		**Transportation**	Car payment	$415	
	Disability Insurance	$150			Gas	$150	
	Pet Insurance	$150			Car maintenance	$35	
				Total necessary expenses:		$2,430	
				Ideal budget (50% of income)		$1,975	
Wants							
Shopping: (clothing, jewelry, decor, etc.)		$100		**Travel**		$200	
Stream-ing services		$50		**Concert tickets**		$150	
Gym membership		$75		**Dining out and bars**		$100	
Hobbies (video games, craft projects)		$165		**Take out**		$200	
				Total wants		$1,040	
				Ideal budget (30% of income)		$1,185	

		Savings		
	Emergency fund (target 30,000)	$150		
	Retire-ment account	$50		
	Other investments	$50		
			Total savings	$250
			Ideal budget (20% of income)	$790
Total expenses:	$3,720			
Net:	$230			

Source: Adapted from Kreisler et al. 2025

CONSUMER DEBT

Managing consumer debt and credit is essential in personal finance. Consumer debt includes credit cards and car loans. A study found 58% of veterinary technicians and assistants carry a credit card balance, higher than the national average of 50% (Volk et al. 2024; Bankrate 2024). Veterinarians also face this issue, especially early in their careers. With interest rates around 22.77%, this debt can add stress, but building adequate savings can help prevent it.

Popular debt repayment methods include the snowball method (paying off the smallest debts first) and the avalanche method (paying off debts with the highest interest rates first). When paying off debt, prioritize consumer debt over student loans. Student loans have a variety of repayment strategies that can lessen their cash flow burden, which will be covered in the next section.

STUDENT DEBT

According to the Merck Wellbeing Study, high levels of student debt are the second-highest risk factor for well-being concerns, and student debt is a common reason cited among veterinarians who would not recommend their profession (Volk et al. 2020, Merck Vet Wellbeing 2023). In 2023, more than 60% of respondents without student debt were flourishing, compared to around 38% of those with $300,000 or more of educational debt (Merck Vet Wellbeing 2024). The mean student debt for 2023 vet school graduates with student loans was $185,486 (Doherty et al. 2024).

Among veterinary technician respondents to the National Association of Veterinary Technicians in America (NAVTA) 2022 Demographic Survey, more than one-third had student debt, with an average of $29,700 among those with debt (NAVTA 2022). Those without student debt had lower burnout and psychological distress (Merck Vet Team Wellbeing 2024). Because veterinary technicians often earn less than other healthcare professionals, managing student debt can be especially challenging.

With numerous student debt resources available to veterinary professionals, there is a path to repayment for everyone, regardless of circumstance. Being intentional about your student loan repayment strategy can give you peace of mind and set you up for success financially. The best approach for you will depend on multiple factors, including your specific numbers and your personal, professional, and financial goals.

Repayment Strategies

The first key distinction in evaluating repayment strategies is the difference between federal and private student loans. Federal loans offer several repayment options, while private loans have only one: paying the balance in full. Because private loans provide little repayment flexibility, students who are still in school should aim to borrow as little as possible.

The One Big Beautiful Bill Act (OBBBA) introduced multiple changes to student loan repayment plans and introduced borrowing limits on federal student loans for graduate and professional students. Graduate PLUS loans, which previously allowed veterinary students to borrow federal student loans up to the full cost of attendance, are set to be eliminated effective July 1, 2026. The law limits professional students (including veterinary students) to borrowing a maximum of $50,000 per year in unsubsidized federal loans, with a total aggregate cap of $200,000. Students enrolled in graduate programs will have a total aggregate cap of $100,000. The borrowing cap applies to students who begin a program of study after July 1, 2026 (One Big Beautiful Bill Act). No changes were made to undergraduate borrowing limits.

When the OBBBA was signed, most veterinary schools already had cost of attendance exceeding the new federal borrowing limits. As a result, many veterinary students will likely need to take out private loans to cover tuition and living expenses. Private student loans typically come with stricter credit requirements and often require a cosigner. This raises concerns about equitable access to veterinary education, since students from lower-income backgrounds or those without access to a qualified cosigner may find it more difficult to attend veterinary school. In addition, private loans usually carry higher interest rates than federal loans, and it remains to be seen whether lenders will adjust their rates and underwriting standards in response to these changes (Singler 2025).

Types of repayment plans for federal student loans include fixed payment plans and income-driven repayment plans. The choice of repayment plans depends on a variety of factors, but a key factor is your debt-to-income ratio, in this case, the ratio between your student debt and your income. Professionals whose student debt greatly exceeds their annual income are more likely to benefit from the passive approach enabled by income-driven repayment plans, rather than an aggressive approach to student loan payoff. A passive approach involves paying only the minimum payment to maximize the benefit of student loan forgiveness. Students and new graduates are often surprised to find out that, depending on their numbers, they may save money overall by paying the minimum income-based payment and going for student loan forgiveness, which we discuss in the next section. These savings may be more impactful once the opportunity cost of diverting cash flow toward retirement savings, home ownership, or other financial goals is considered.

A common mistake we see is professionals who pay extra toward their student loans while going for forgiveness, rather than committing to a passive repayment strategy. Paying more than the minimum payment is not beneficial if you are planning for forgiveness, since you would be paying on debt that would otherwise be forgiven. Extra cash flow is better directed toward other financial goals or saving for the potential tax bill due at the end of forgiveness.

In contrast, professionals with student debt lower than their annual income will likely pay the loans to zero; thus, they may decide to pay off aggressively (e.g. to save money on interest over the life of the loan) or more passively (e.g. to free up funds for other financial goals). If an aggressive repayment strategy has been selected, there can be advantages to paying extra. Payments that exceed the required monthly payment should be applied to the loan principal, which can typically be specified on the loan servicer's website when the payment is made to prevent the money from being applied to future interest.

Fixed payment plans include Standard repayment plans that range from 10 to 25 years, depending on the initial student loan balance, or up to 30 years for consolidated loans. A Standard repayment plan has a fixed monthly payment based on how much you owe and your interest rate. For many veterinary professionals, payments on the Standard plan are too high to be affordable.

There are a variety of income-based repayment strategies, which are summarized in Table 8.3. Due to legal challenges, what payment plans are available and their exact terms has been a shifting landscape since the pandemic. Moreover, a multitude of individual factors contribute to finding the right repayment strategy. Therefore, it is recommended that you use an up-to-date student loan calculator and references when choosing a repayment strategy, such as those found through the VIN Foundation (https://vinfoundation.org/resources/veterinary-student-debt/) or Student Loan Planner (https://www.studentloanplanner.com). It is also prudent to seek the advice of a Certified Student Loan Professional (CSLP®) when deciding which plan fits your individual situation. In Story 8.1, two veterinarians explain how student loans impacted their lives until they settled on a repayment strategy.

Upon graduation, federal student loans enter a six-month grace period, during which no payments are required. For new graduates pursuing student loan forgiveness, consolidating loans through StudentAid.gov has historically been a valuable strategy. Consolidation allows borrowers to end the grace period early and start progress toward forgiveness on an income-driven repayment plan. Because most students have little to no income the year before graduation, initial income-driven payments are often calculated between \$0 and \$10 per month. For those with Health Professions Student Loans, federal consolidation can also make these loans eligible for forgiveness by combining them with Direct Loans (Consolidating Student Loans FSA 2024).

Table 8.3 Income-driven repayment plans.

	Payment term (years)	Payments based on	Notes
Repayment Assistance Plan (RAP)	30	Up to 10% of income	Unpaid interest is subsidized and therefore overall loan balance does not increase. Based on 10% of income if Adjusted Gross Income (AGI) is >$100k, with a sliding scale if AGI <$100k. May be the only income-driven plan available for those who borrow loans after July 1, 2026.
Income Based Repayment (IBR) – New	20	10% of discretionary income	Available to borrowers who began borrowing loans between July 1, 2014, and June 30, 2026. Those who borrow loans on or after July 1, 2026, are ineligible.
Income Based Repayment (IBR) – Old	25	15% of discretionary income	Available to borrowers with an outstanding balance before July 1, 2014. Those who borrow loans on or after July 1, 2026, are ineligible.
Saving on a Valuable Education (SAVE)	20–25	10% of discretionary income	To be phased out between July 2026 and 2028
Pay As You Earn (PAYE)	20	10% of discretionary income	To be phased out between July 2026 and 2028
Income-Contingent Repayment (ICR)	25	20% of discretionary income or an income-adjusted fixed 12-year repayment plan	To be phased out between July 2026 and 2028

STORY 8.1 STUDENT LOANS

Story A: Payoff strategy

The feeling of overwhelm from student debt caused me to postpone life stages like marriage/children, caused me to get three jobs and work 7 days a week for 2.5 years, to finally feel like I was making headway on my loans. It was a terrible time in my life, full of anxiety and stress and feeling like it would never get better. I did however buy a house, which just happened to be a good time to do so in my region, which has since boomed (bought in 2017). Honestly the pandemic interest rate pause was the best thing that could ever happened to me. I started investing in the stock market, I started contributing larger chunks to my loans, and once the interest pause ended, it put the fire under my bum to just pay them off. The gains from my stocks helped pay them off too. Finally, 10 years after graduation they are paid off and it is great. I hope the higher salaries of vets these days helps people get ahead a little faster, but I know cost of living is so high in many places, the feeling of hopelessness is hard not to feel. I think really writing everything out and setting goals for each year is what will keep you motivated to keep chipping away, or paying minimums for forgiveness, whatever plan makes most sense. I got so burnt-out working 60–70+ hours a week for 2.5 years that I can only work 3–4 days a week these days, and I take my life much slower. Luckily, I own my own business now and am financially stable without overworking.

Story B: Income-based repayment strategy

As an aspiring practice owner, I knew I had to have a game plan for my home-sized student loans. I discussed my goal with a financial advisor, and with my professional goals in mind, we made a plan. For me, using an income-based repayment plan has allowed me to save additional finances to build the career of my dreams. Without this plan, I would not be able to have a sizable down payment for the practice I will be purchasing. I have a clear vision for managing my student loans without them negatively impacting how I want my life to develop. For my story, using the opportunity of forgiveness has opened doors for financial success that far outweigh paying off my loans at a breakneck pace. I think more people should learn to leverage debt as an opportunity to increase wealth—many successful people have used this model. Also, my large student debt did not negatively impact my practice purchase financing approval for a multi-million-dollar practice purchase.

Since consolidation rules—and repayment plan eligibility for consolidated loans—may change in the future, borrowers should consult up-to-date resources from the VIN Foundation (https://vinfoundation.org/resources/veterinary-student-debt/) or seek guidance from a Certified Student Loan Professional (CSLP®) before consolidating. Notably, consolidations completed after July 1, 2026, will limit repayment options to the Repayment Assistance Plan (RAP) or Standard repayment plan only, according to the One Big Beautiful Bill Act.

Note that federal consolidation is very different from private refinancing. With federal consolidation, student loans remain eligible for income-driven repayment plans and forgiveness. With refinancing, federal student loans become private loans and lose these benefits. Federal student loans should not be refinanced without first consulting a student loan professional. For private student loans, refinancing may provide a lower interest rate and more favorable payment terms.

Loan Forgiveness and Debt Relief Programs

Through income-driven repayment plans, student loan forgiveness is available to veterinary professionals regardless of job type or sector. On income-driven plans, the student loan balance is forgiven after 20–30 years of payments and is considered to be taxable income the year the loans are forgiven. This tax implication, often called the tax bomb, is an important part of financial planning for veterinary professionals who are pursuing long-term forgiveness. Financial planners recommend saving for the tax bomb by making recurring deposits into a brokerage account (nonretirement investment account). The American Rescue Plan Act of 2021 included a provision that made forgiven or discharged student loan debt tax-free between December 31, 2020, and January 1, 2026 (Payment Count Adjustment FSA 2024). Although some experts have speculated that a similar law or provision may become available in the future, it is prudent to be prepared for the tax bomb.

Veterinarians who work 30 hours per week or more in a nonprofit or government role can become eligible for Public Service Loan Forgiveness (PSLF) after 10 years of qualifying payments on their federal student loans. PSLF forgiveness is tax-free at the federal level. Veterinary professionals who are pursuing PSLF should enroll in an income-driven repayment plan to maximize their opportunity for student loan forgiveness. Annual employment certification is recommended to document eligibility and progress toward PSLF.

The Veterinary Medicine Loan Repayment Program pays up to $40,000 per year towards qualified student loans for veterinarians who agree to serve in shortage areas designated by the National Institute of Food and Agriculture for a three-year period. Additional payments are made to participants to offset the federal taxes associated with the income from this program (USDA 2024). Some states offer their own student loan repayment or forgiveness programs for service in underserved areas.

INVESTMENTS AND RETIREMENT

Investing is the process of putting money into assets like stocks, bonds, or real estate with the expectation that it will grow over time. Establishing a habit of investing early in your career, even with small amounts, can make a significant difference by the time you retire. Compound interest, where the returns on your investments generate even more returns, makes early and consistent investing a powerful tool for financial growth. Table 8.4 shows three scenarios of investment: that of a person who invests a small amount into the stock market monthly starting at age 25 years, the same investments starting at age 45 years, and the comparative contribution that it would take to reach a similar final balance.

Of course, the stock market can change from day to day, and having all your proverbial eggs in one basket could lead to a bad scenario should the market crash just as you need access to these investments. Having a diversified portfolio—one that spreads investments across different asset types—can help manage risk and increase the likelihood of steady growth. While investing involves some level of uncertainty, careful planning can offer veterinary professionals peace of mind and financial independence over time.

Table 8.4 Reported benefits by role.

Benefit type	Veterinarians	Technicians
Paid vacation leave	69% overall; 67% in private practice; 77% in public practice	75% offered paid time off; 41% use all allotted time; 9% receive none
Paid sick leave	58% overall, highest in public practice	Often combined with general paid time off; dedicated sick leave less common
Medical or health insurance	68% overall; 70% in public practice; 65% in private practice	Offered by approximately 46% of employers
Continuing education (CE) expenses	75% overall; 78% in private practice; 63% in public practice	72% report CE support or reimbursement
Professional licenses or association dues	74% license coverage; 66% dues coverage	55% employer support for licensing or credential fees
Discounted pet care	64% overall; 72% in private practice	80% report access to pet care discounts
Retirement plan (e.g. 401k)	64% overall, higher in corporate and public sectors	39% report access to retirement savings plans
Mental health or employee assistance programs (EAPs)	48% overall, rising among large employers	46% have access to an assistance program
Student debt relief	22% of employers contribute to repayment or PSLF support	16% report employer-sponsored debt relief

Source: AVMA (2025); NAVTA (2024).

When planning for investments, it's wise to utilize retirement accounts as part of your strategy. An employer retirement plan, like a 401k, 403b, or Simple IRA, allows you to make regular investments in your future by contributing directly from your paychecks. Often, these plans will have a plan administrator, who may help guide the investments. Pretax contributions to employer retirement accounts have tax advantages and can lower student loan payments for those on income-driven repayment plans. Your employer may also make contributions to these accounts as a match to your contribution or as a flat contribution, which will increase your investment. Individual retirement accounts (IRAs) and Roth IRAs are retirement accounts that are opened by individuals through a broker or bank, and they often have a wider array of investment options compared with employer plans. Each retirement account type has an annual contribution limit, and IRAs and Roth IRAs are subject to rules about tax treatment and eligibility. A full discussion of this topic is beyond the scope of this book. Investopedia.com provides up-to-date resources on retirement planning and investing (Investopedia n.d.).

SAVINGS AND INSURANCE

When planning for financial stability, some thought must be given to the unexpected. Things like illness, injury, and property damage can be financially devastating without adequate planning. Two tools help us plan for the unexpected: savings and insurance.

An emergency fund is a foundational component of any financial plan, providing a cushion to absorb any major changes to your monthly cash flow. Unplanned expenses are a part of life, and insufficient savings is a common reason for credit card debt.

There are two levels of emergency fund: (1) a starter fund and (2) savings of three to six months of expenses. A starter emergency fund of $3,000–$5,000 provides a foundation that will give you peace of mind that you'll be able to handle many unexpected expenses that may arise. Once you have your starter fund, the next goal is to save three to six months of basic living expenses. This amount of savings will allow you to navigate more significant financial emergencies, such as income loss due to

Table 8.5 Compound interest.

Age at starting investment	25	45	45
Monthly contribution	$200.00	$200.00	$1,551.00
Balance at retirement	$1,114,596	$144,325	$1,114,693

Source: Forbes Advisor. (2024); NerdWallet. (2024).

job loss or disability. Setting up automatic transfers to a high-yield savings account is a great way to build your emergency fund.

Insurance is another tool that can help maintain financial stability during unexpected events. It prevents financial hardship by covering costs that could otherwise drain savings or lead to debt. A list of common types of insurance is available in Table 8.5.

Disability insurance is particularly important in veterinary medicine, which consistently ranks among the top five most dangerous professions for nonfatal illness and injury according to the Occupational Safety and Health Administration (Bureau of Labor Statistics 2023). Long-term disability coverage provides income protection if an injury prevents work for an extended period, helping maintain financial security. Short-term disability insurance can also be important, particularly for individuals who plan to have children. It offers income replacement during maternity leave, ensuring financial stability during recovery and easing the transition back to work. The easiest time to qualify for disability insurance is early in your career, as illnesses and injuries over time can lead to policy exclusions and denials. Guaranteed Standard Issue (GSI) disability insurance policies may be available for final-year veterinary students or newly graduated veterinarians who can lock in favorable rates without medical underwriting. For example, the AVMA offers disability insurance to third- and fourth-year veterinary students, as well as to recent graduates (<60 days), through its Graduate Guarantee Acceptance Program, with no required medical history review or exams. Veterinary technicians or experienced veterinarians can purchase a policy on the open market or through a professional association.

Professional liability insurance is crucial for veterinarians as it protects against legal claims of malpractice, providing financial coverage for legal fees and settlements. License defense insurance is equally important, safeguarding veterinarians by covering the costs associated with defending their professional license in the event of a complaint or investigation.

COMPENSATION AND WELL-BEING

COMPENSATION MODELS

Compensation models for veterinary professionals vary between and within job roles in the clinic. The most common pay structure for veterinary support staff is hourly. Some support staff may be paid on a salary basis, but they should be aware of the federal and state laws applicable to their role regarding salary, hours, and overtime. Salaried employees are categorized as either exempt from overtime pay or nonexempt. The Federal Labor Standards Act states that, unless employees are exempt, they must be paid overtime. Exempt employees are not paid overtime and are generally defined by several criteria, including a salary level, management duties, the need for independent work, and the need for advanced degrees and licenses to perform said work (U.S. Department of Labor 2019).

Compensation structures for veterinarians are more variable. The most common compensation structure is a straight salary or a combination of salary and production pay. Hourly or shift pay is more common for relief veterinarians, although shift pay may be part of the compensation structure for some small-animal emergency practices. Straight production, where compensation is based solely on commission with no guaranteed minimum, is uncommon. A 2023 survey of new graduate veterinarians found that 68.8% accepted a position with a base salary plus production, and 30.9% accepted a guaranteed salary-only position (Doherty et al. 2024).

Production-based compensation for veterinarians has been the subject of a lively debate among veterinary professionals over the past several years (Hauser and Fuhrman 2018; Zakharenkov 2023; Lau 2023). Some veterinarians believe production-based compensation encourages a strong work ethic or a greater appreciation for the business side of veterinary practice. On the other hand, some veterinarians feel that production-based pay may negatively impact well-being or practice culture. Some are concerned that vets may be discouraged from taking vacation (since they won't be producing during time off), or that production pay drives increased patient numbers and therefore overwork, and could incentivize veterinarians to inflate the client's bill or encourage unhealthy competition (Hauser and Fuhrman 2018; Steffey et al. 2023; Zakharenkov 2023). Story 8.2 shares the stories of two veterinarians and their different perspectives on compensation models.

In the Merck Veterinary Wellbeing Study, satisfaction with compensation is a predictor of high well-being and positive mental health among veterinarians (Volk et al. 2020). In this study, compensation structure was found not to be a significant factor in job satisfaction. However, satisfaction with the method of compensation was lower for veterinarians on a straight salary, and salary was negatively associated with burnout (Volk et al. 2020). These findings are, however, not consistent across studies. For example, production-based compensation has been associated with higher levels of burnout in physicians and can also exacerbate moral distress, as the needs of patients may conflict with the business aspects of practice (Steffey et al. 2023).

BENEFITS

Another aspect of compensation are benefits, including things like health care, CE, license and association fees. Table 8.6 lists benefits commonly offered in veterinary jobs. While benefits have a notable impact on total compensation, their link to well-being is once again complex. For instance, in a 2023 survey, veterinarians preferred working in private vs corporate practice (55% vs 12%),

STORY 8.2 IMPACTS OF PRODUCTION VS SALARY

Story A: A veterinarian who prefers salary compensation

I am in small animal general practice, four years post-grad. When I worked base + production, there was a constant pressure from higher-ups to produce more. There was competition between doctors to get the more expensive cases. I felt like I wasn't able to offer a spectrum of care (spectrum of care meaning discussing gold standard, but working with cost-concerned clients to do the next best thing). Now I'm on salary and I love it. I don't feel pressured to work harder/longer or to push things on clients. I don't care that I potentially could make more if I was paid a different way than salary. I'm able to personalize the medicine to the specific client and pet based on their needs.

Story B: A veterinarian who prefers production-based compensation

I work ER. We all remember how bad the pandemic was. Twenty ERs within driving distance, and at any given time usually less than five of them were open to new cases. It wasn't uncommon for every single ER's status to be listed as closed. If a stable patient waited less than four hours to be seen, we were doing awesome. Like most of us, I was working at maximum capacity every day. If I'd been on salary, I would have been paid the exact same amount. Instead, my already high income went up by 50% from 2019 to 2020, and has stayed permanently higher. I didn't have to wait months for my review, justify myself, and maneuver through a negotiation; I just got paid what I was worth. Seeing such a direct connection between how hard I work and how much money I take home, for me, makes it much easier to stay motivated as a veterinarian.

Anonymous veterinarian

Table 8.6 Types of insurance.

	Description
Medical	
EPO	Except in an emergency, only covered if in network*. Specialty care does not require referral.
HMO	Except in an emergency, only covered if in network*. Specialty care does require referral.
POS	Patients pay less when seeing in network providers. Specialty care does require a referral.
PPO	Patients pay less when seeing in network providers. Specialty care does not require a referral.
Disability	
Short Term	Provides income replacement for a limited period of time, often less than six months.
Long term	After a waiting period, provides long-term income replacement lasting a fixed number of years or until retirement.
Life	
Term	Provides a benefit during a specific period of time, usually between 10 and 30 years
Whole	Provides a benefit lasting entire life. Premiums are fixed. Portion of premiums are placed into cash value account
Universal	Provides a benefit lasting entire life. Premiums are flexible. Portion of premiums are placed into cash value account
Professional liability	Protects against claims of malpractice or negligence in professional services.
License defense	Covers legal costs for defending a professional license during investigations or complaints.
Auto insurance	Covers damages and liability for car accidents or theft.
Homeowners/renters	Covers property damage, theft, and liability in homes or rental units.
Umbrella	Provides additional liability coverage beyond standard policies.

* "In Network" refers to a group of hospitals, doctors, pharmacies and other service providers that have a contract with the insurance company.

Source: Adapted from https://www.healthcare.gov/choose-a-plan/plan-types

despite corporate veterinarians reporting better access to benefits (Kogan 2023). While this study shows that benefits alone do not fully explain job satisfaction, benefits can still indirectly impact well-being. For instance, professional development and access to CE has been linked to well-being across veterinary team members (Cake et al. 2015; Kogan et al. 2020). Therefore, a benefit like a CE budget can have an indirect positive impact on well-being.

OTHER CONTRACT TERMS

Noncompetes and signing bonuses are other factors to consider when evaluating job opportunities. Some practices require associates to sign a noncompete clause as a condition of employment, which may affect finances indirectly by limiting opportunities to moonlight at other practices (Morello 2023). This concern can be mitigated by reducing the scope of practice, timeframe, or mileage associated with the noncompete, or eliminated by finding a practice that does not require one. As of this writing, a Federal Trade Commission rule banning noncompetes is facing court challenges (FTC 2024). A signing bonus may be appealing, but may come with a stipulation that it must be paid back if the individual leaves before a certain timeframe has passed. Additionally, because the bonus is taxed when received and repayment amounts are usually based on the total

STORY 8.3 SIGNING BONUSES

Story A

I took a sizable bonus for a medical director job at a one to two doctor corporate practice in August 2022. I spent a large chunk of it on a bucket list two-month Danube river cruise with my wife. It was a magical time, and I wouldn't trade that for anything. However, I was tied to a year of service with the company or would've owed the full amount back. Unfortunately, it ended up being a bad fit for a number of reasons. Three or four months in, I was looking for a way out. I approached a couple of privately owned practices where I had worked relief in the past, and none were willing to buy out my contract.

I stuck with the job for 20 months total in the end. I stayed those extra months because of some quarterly and year-end bonuses that were coming up, as well as guilt about leaving my patients and team without a doctor. That period of time was the worst mental health time of my career. It was the first time I'd ever considered leaving clinical practice entirely.

Story B

I took a $10k signing bonus. The clinic offered to apply it to the principal of my loans, but I didn't have any loans, so I took it as income (and paid income taxes). $5k at signing and $5k after 30 days. Claw-back clause in the contract stated I had to pay back the whole $10k if I didn't fulfill 12 months (quit or fired). I have enjoyed my first year here and looking forward to more, and now that I'm past the point of having to pay it back, I'm glad I did it. It helped cover moving expenses and set up an emergency fund if my housing or car situation ran into trouble.

Anonymous veterinarian

pretax amount, the amount owed back can exceed what was originally received. As discussed in Story 8.3, this may leave someone financially tied to a practice they do not enjoy working in. Asking for a prorated repayment provision in the contract reduces the risk of having to repay the entire bonus (Roasa 2022).

CONTRACT NEGOTIATION

Despite a strong job market, many veterinarians do not negotiate their initial offer. Surveys of new graduates suggest that only about one-third negotiate, even though employers report willingness to adjust salary, benefits, or scheduling (Taylor 2018; Allen 2016). Gender dynamics also influence negotiation outcomes. Although women now constitute the majority of the profession, men continue to earn higher average incomes, including salary differences of up to $100,000 in the highest-earning quartile (Neill et al., 2021). A 2023 review found that women negotiate less frequently and may anticipate greater social or professional backlash when they do, contributing to persistent wage gaps (Vesterlund and Recalde 2023). These inequities are not solely an individual's responsibility to solve. In 2016, an AVMA salary calculator drew criticism for applying a built-in deduction for women based on historical earnings data. This serves as a reminder that negotiation landscapes are shaped not only by personal behavior, but also by how compensation norms and tools reflect and perpetuate structural inequities (Silverman 2016). After criticism, the AVMA calculator no longer considers gender when calculating salaries. This change is an example of how organizational-level systems can affect workplace equity.

In general, veterinary support staff rarely receive formal contracts. However, many receive offer letters, which provide a similar opportunity for negotiation and clarification. Even without a formal document, a clear discussion of terms benefits both employees and employers. Table 8.7 highlights practical steps that support fair compensation, clarity, and long-term well-being in employment agreements.

Table 8.7 The following are tips on how to best negotiate an employment contract.

Successful contract negotiation:
Clarify expectations and compensation structure
Contracts should define how an employee will be paid and what duties they are responsible for. For production-based pay, it is important to know what counts toward production, how time off affects income, and whether discounts or write-offs apply (Ervasti 2023 2023; Zoetis 2024). Other expectations, such as emergency or weekend coverage, should also be specified to avoid later conflict (Mandelbaum Barrett 2023).
Get professional help reviewing terms
Many veterinarians sign their first contract without legal review, but small wording differences can have major consequences. Attorneys familiar with veterinary employment can identify unusual clauses, especially around production pay, malpractice coverage, and bonus repayment (Mandelbaum Barrett 2023; Zoetis 2024). The cost of review is often outweighed by long-term financial protection (Davidow 2018).
Communicate professionally and collaboratively
Negotiation is not adversarial. Approaching discussions with clarity and flexibility supports a positive working relationship (DVM360 2016). Prioritizing key concerns and proposing solutions that work for both parties can lead to better agreements and practice culture (Vet Idealist 2018; Zoetis 2024).
Verbal promises are not enforceable
Any negotiated changes must be written into the final contract (Mandelbaum Barrett 2023). If it is not written, it does not exist. Confirming the final document reflects all agreed-upon terms protects both parties from misunderstanding (Zoetis 2024).
Restrictive clauses and separation terms
Noncompete and nonsolicitation agreements can limit future employment options. Important details include geographic radius, duration, and whether restrictions apply across multiple locations (Mandelbaum Barrett 2023). Narrowing the radius, timeframe, or scope may provide a workable compromise (Zoetis 2024). Contracts should also specify notice periods and how final pay or production bonuses are handled. Some bonuses must be repaid if an employee leaves early, often based on the pretax amount (Roasa 2022).

PRACTICE OWNERSHIP

Owning a practice is a career choice that offers greater autonomy at work and often leads to higher well-being. The Merck Well-being Study found that 23% of associates experienced high burnout, compared to just 11% of practice owners (Merck Vet Wellbeing 2024). Additionally, practice owners report higher job satisfaction, with 83.4% satisfied, compared to 63.9% of associates (Doherty et al. 2024).

Autonomy is not the only benefit of ownership, as it can also have financial rewards. Practice owners have higher income potential and build an asset that increases in value. In 2023, owners earned an average of $180,728, compared to $135,259 for associates (Doherty et al. 2024). In Story 8.4, a veterinarian details how they have benefited from practice ownership.

There are several pathways to practice ownership, each offering different levels of control and financial investment. Independently owned practices provide veterinarians with full management authority and decision-making autonomy. These include *de novo* practices, which are clinics built from the ground up. Starting a practice in this way can be rewarding but requires significant time and financial commitment. Buy-ins and buyouts offer opportunities to purchase partial or full ownership of an existing hospital, providing a smoother transition with established systems and clientele (Keiser 2021).

STORY 8.4 A HAPPY PRACTICE OWNER

I knew from a very young age that I wanted to be a veterinarian. I also knew pretty early on in my college years that I wanted to own a practice. I was drawn to the business aspect as well as the medicine. My first ownership experience was a mobile practice that I took great pride in, but wasn't as profitable for multiple reasons. I then thought that I wanted to partner in a big practice. I thought it sounded better to be a collaborative business partner. . .less risk and greater reward. The opportunity then slapped me across the face to become a solo practice owner of a practice that I knew had great potential. Three years into making that leap, I am very proud of what I have built, both from the business and human relations aspects. My financial successes will afford me an overall better life, while still supporting my community. My biggest headache is also one of my greatest accomplishments, and that is the people part. Practice ownership has helped me become and will continue to push me to be a better person, leader, human. While maybe not in the best way, or most "correct" way, I have helped others (my employees) become better humans with fantastic skills. We all will continue to learn together. We all will continue to make mistakes together, but I am happier and more satisfied with my career and myself, overall because I became a practice owner.

Corporate partnership models present alternative ownership options for those seeking shared equity with reduced administrative responsibility. In a joint venture, veterinarians typically hold a minority equity stake in their practice, while the corporation maintains majority ownership and manages operations. Other arrangements allow veterinarians to share in equity ownership across a network of hospitals. These models may appeal to those who value financial participation without the full management burden, or who are preparing to transition out of private ownership (Lewandowski 2024). However, such partnerships often provide less autonomy and decision latitude than traditional independent ownership.

The veterinarian in Story 8.5, discusses the pros and cons they experienced as both a private owner and as a minority shareholder.

CAREER PATH AND WELL-BEING

While ownership offers autonomy and potential financial rewards, it is only one of many professional pathways within veterinary medicine. For those seeking different challenges or work–life balance, a variety of alternative career paths exist for both veterinarians and veterinary staff.

VETERINARIANS

Rising incomes and a focus on well-being in veterinary medicine have sparked discussions on how career choices affect financial well-being. A study of veterinarians from 2001 to 2021 found that graduates with higher student debt were more likely to pursue higher-paying positions or advanced education (Bain and Lefebvre 2022). Those same graduates were less likely to enter public practice, despite the availability of PSLF programs (Bain and Lefebvre 2022).

In the past, seeking mentorship often meant accepting lower pay through internships or residencies. Recently, however, structured mentorship programs within private practices have emerged, allowing new graduates to gain professional guidance while earning an associate-level salary (McPhetridge et al. 2022; Morello 2023). Postdoctoral certificate programs in areas such as acupuncture and physical rehabilitation also offer advanced training and expanded career opportunities. Most are structured to accommodate full-time employment during completion.

STORY 8.5 EXPERIENCES AS A SOLO OWNER AND SHAREHOLDER

Practice ownership is a delicate balance. You want to serve your patients, your clients, you want to be "the cool fun boss," and at the end of the day you also need to run a profitable business. That last one is I think particularly hard for vets. I thought after 34 years, I had a pretty good handle on the industry. I was still unprepared for ownership. I was unprepared because I did not have the personality type that allowed me to capably and confidently confront the demands of the financial decisions that needed to be made, the management issues, the social media management, and the medical director position that is needed when you have multiple doctors on staff. Never mind actually being a doctor!

I strongly believe that some people are mentally able to be either the chef or the sous chef. And often you don't know which category you fall into until you try on all of the hats. I realized within two years of ownership I was mentally unable to wear the big hat alone. I tried an independent management contractor. They were helpful, but it wasn't enough. I continued to work all hours of the day and still felt like an imposter. I felt like I was failing everyone. So, I turned to someone to solve all the problems that are related to the business side of things: the corporate entity. Like so many other vets, I was drawn in by the promise that they would handle the business side of things, and I could just return to being a vet. So I sold my company. I would still be a co-owner, albeit with a minority of shares, and they would slowly buy me out over the next three years.

Initially, my corporate buyout was a wonderful collaboration. Lots of big promises were made, but at the end of the day, business people really care about business. Judgment by spreadsheet comes into play. The competition begins amongst the clinics in the company's portfolio, and profitability becomes the watchword. What I thought would be a stress reliever became the most stressful time of my life. The previous concerns of failure were compounded 100-fold, and I got into a very dangerous place mental health wise. Thankfully, I got some help, and I was slightly more prepared to handle the judgment of my business partners and, therefore, was able to make a plan to extract myself from ownership. The task I had set for myself at the beginning was not meant to be.

My experiences taught me that the mix of business and an empathy-driven field like veterinary medicine is a very delicate balance. To sail those waters successfully takes a rare and skilled person. I have met and conversed with a few of those rare singularities. All of them are veterinarians first and foremost. I'm not sure corporate entities are capable of understanding the heart of this profession, yet they are for many lost souls the only life raft they can see. I truly hope for our profession, we can find a better solution where like-minded people can collaborate and focus on the profession we all love.

For those pursuing board certification, financial trade-offs remain significant. Advanced training typically involves years of reduced income, and concerns are growing that debt-to-income ratios and low stipends for house officers are discouraging veterinarians from pursuing academic careers, potentially contributing to shortages of veterinary educators (Lairmore 2024). Salaries for interns and residents continue to lag behind those in private practice (McPhetridge et al. 2022; Morello et al. 2021; Doherty et al. 2024). A 2021 analysis found that many training programs paid below a living wage, though a 2023 follow-up reported modest improvements (Morello et al. 2021; Morello 2023).

Financial pressure, extended work hours, and limited opportunities for self-care during training all contribute to high stress levels—over 95% of house officers report financial anxiety (McPhetridge et al. 2022). Yet despite these challenges, more than half of trainees (55%) believed the experience was worth the financial sacrifice (AAVMC 2020). Specialists ultimately tend to earn higher incomes than general practitioners, though compensation varies by specialty and practice type. In 2023, specialists reported an average income of $226,293, compared with $137,017 for general practitioners (Doherty et al. 2024).

SUPPORT STAFF

Career development is closely linked to well-being for veterinary support staff. From assistant to technician and beyond, access to structured growth opportunities provides a sense of competence and stability in a demanding field. Studies show that technicians value the ability to apply their skills and to be recognized for their work, but many report limited advancement and inconsistent utilization (Kogan et al. 2020; Reinhard et al. 2025). The 2024 Merck Animal Health Veterinary Team Study found that nonveterinarian staff experienced similar burnout levels to veterinarians, but higher financial stress and twice the rate of serious psychological distress (Volk et al. 2024). These findings indicate that well-being for support staff depends not only on emotional resilience but also on adequate compensation and meaningful career progression.

Education and certification are important drivers of both satisfaction and pay. Credentialed technicians with higher degrees earn more: those with associate degrees averaged $19.93 per hour, compared with $22.37 for bachelor's and $27.55 for master's degree holders (Gilliam and Coates 2020). Veterinary Technician Specialists (VTSs) also reported benefits: 76% received a raise after certification, though most salary increases were modest, typically less than 10% (Kogan et al. 2025). Many specialists described the underutilization of their training and unclear role boundaries, suggesting that professional credentials alone do not guarantee improved working conditions.

Career transitions into teaching, research, or management can improve retention and well-being by providing greater autonomy and defined responsibilities. Turnover rates among veterinary technicians have historically been high, reaching 33% annually in some institutions, but retention improves when staff have access to advancement, ongoing education, and recognition for certification (Huerkamp 2006). Those who progress into educational or supervisory positions often report more predictable schedules and higher job satisfaction. However, such roles remain limited and may require financial or institutional support for additional training.

Demographic and economic factors also influence well-being. Lower pay, limited benefits, and systemic inequities contribute to financial stress and psychological strain among client service representatives, assistants, and technicians (Scoresby et al. 2023). Expanding access to career development, improving pay equity, and increasing the effective use of credentialed technicians are practical strategies to reduce burnout and strengthen the veterinary workforce. When staff have clear and supported paths for growth, studies show improvements in retention and professional well-being, and evidence from high-stakes tasks like anesthesia suggests these advancements also contribute to safer, higher-quality patient care (Kogan et al. 2020; Kogan et al. 2025; Reinhard et al. 2025).

CONCLUSION

Financial well-being is an essential part of a sustainable and fulfilling veterinary career. Understanding money not only reduces stress but also creates space for choice, autonomy, and meaning in work and life. When financial plans align with personal values and professional goals, they support both stability and the sense of purpose that drew many into the field in the first place.

REFERENCES

10 Questions to Ask Your Financial Advisor. *CFP Board.* https://www.letsmakeaplan.org/choosing-a-planner/10-questions-to-ask-your-financial-advisor (accessed 4 October 2024).

American Veterinary Medical Association (AVMA) (2025). Managing personal finances. https://www.avma.org/resources-tools/personal-finance (accessed 14 December 2025).

Archuleta, K., Asebedo, S., and Palmer, L. (2019). Contemporary theories and frameworks for use in financial counseling. In: *Financial Counseling* (ed. D. Durband, R. Law, and A. Mazzolini), 103–104.

Bain, B. and Lefebvre, S. (2022). Associations between career choice and educational debt for fourth-year students of US veterinary schools and colleges,

2001–2021. *Journal of the American Veterinary Medical Association* 260 (9): 1064–1068.

Bankrate, 2024. Survey: Half of American cardholders now carry credit card debt, many with no plan to pay it off. https://www.bankrate.com/credit-cards/news/credit-card-debt-survey/ (accessed 14 December 2025).

Cake, M.A., Bell, M.A., Bickley, N., and Bartram, D.J. (2015). The life of meaning: a model of the positive contributions to well-being from veterinary work. *Journal of Veterinary Medical Education 42* (3): 184–193.

Carr, M.M. and Greenhill, L.M. (2015). Veterinary school applicants: financial literacy and behaviors. *Journal of Veterinary Medical Education 42* (2): 89–96.

Consolidating Student Loans. *Federal Student Aid*. https://studentaid.gov/manage-loans/consolidation (accessed 4 October 2024).

Davidow, B. (2018). Lean in, negotiate, and ask these questions about your veterinary contract. *The Veterinary Idealist*, 22 March. Available at: https://vetidealist.com/negotiate-veterinary-contract/ (accessed 20 April 2026).

Department of Labor (2019). https://www.dol.gov/agencies/whd/fact-sheets/17a-overtime

Doherty, C., McKay, C., and Ouedraogo, F. (2024). *AVMA Report on the Economic State of the Veterinary Profession*. American Veterinary Medical Association.

Ervasti, J. (2023). Mastering the art of veterinary employment contracts. *R^2 Financial Strategies*, 17 October. Available at: https://www.r2fin.com/blog/mastering-the-art-of-veterinary-employment-contracts (accessed 20 April 2026).

Federal Trade Commission (FTC) (2024). FTC announces rule banning noncompetes. https://www.ftc.gov/news-events/news/press-releases/2024/04/ftc-announces-rule-banning-noncompetes (accessed 14 December 2025).

Forbes Advisor. (2024). Investing. *Forbes Advisor*. Available at: https://www.forbes.com/advisor/investing/ Opens a new window (accessed 20 April 2026).

Gilliam, L. and Coates, J.R. (2020). Compensation and benefits for credentialed veterinary technicians in the United States. *Journal of the American Veterinary Medical Association* 256 (11): 1205–1211. https://doi.org/10.2460/javma.256.11.1205.

Hauser, W. and Fuhrman, J. (2018). A prescription for change. *Today's Veterinary Business*, Oct/Nov 2018.

Huerkamp, M.J. (2006). Job dynamics of veterinary professionals in an academic research institution. I. Retention and turnover of veterinary technicians. *Journal of the American Association for Laboratory Animal Science 45* (5): 16–25.

Investopedia (n.d.). Investopedia. https://www.investopedia.com/ (accessed 7 December 2025).

Jebb, A.T., Tay, L., Diener, E., and Oishi, S. (2018). Happiness, income satiation and turning points around the world. *Nature Human Behaviour 2* (1): 33–38.

Kaiser, T. and Menkhoff, L. (2017). Does financial education impact financial literacy and financial behavior, and if so, when? *The World Bank Economic Review* 31 (3): 611–630.

Keiser, S. (2021). Follow the money. *Today's Veterinary Business*, April/May, 2021.

Killingsworth, M.A. (2021). Experienced well-being rises with income, even above $75,000 per year. *Proceedings of the National Academy of Sciences 118* (4): e2016976118.

Kogan, L. and Rishniw, M. (2023). Differences in perceptions and satisfaction exist among veterinarians employed at corporate versus privately owned veterinary clinics. *Journal of the American Veterinary Medical Association* 261 (12): 1838–1846.

Kogan, L.R., Wallace, J.E., Schoenfeld-Tacher, R. et al. (2020). Veterinary technicians and occupational burnout. *Frontiers in Veterinary Science 7*: 328.

Kreisler, R.E., Spindel, M.E., and Rishniw, M. (2025). 2024 Analysis of compensation, job duties, and benefits among US shelter medicine veterinarians. *Journal of the American Veterinary Medical Association 263* (4): 1–9.

Lairmore, M. (2024). An imminent need for veterinary medical educators: are we facing a crisis? *Journal of the American Veterinary Medical Association* 262 (8): 1124–1128.

Lau, E. (2023). How to pay veterinarians: salary, hourly, or on production? *VIN News Service*. https://news.vin.com/default.aspx?pid=210&Id=11653194&f5=1 (accessed 28 July 2024).

Liss, D.J., Kerl, M.E., and Tsai, C.L. (2020). Factors associated with job satisfaction and engagement among credentialed small animal veterinary technicians in the United States. *Journal of the American Veterinary Medical Association 257* (5): 537–545.

Mandelbaum Barrett PC (2023). Unleashing the secrets of veterinary associate contracts, 14 November. Available at: Mandelbaum Barrett website (accessed 20 April 2026).

McPhetridge, J., Scharf, V., Dickson, R., and Thieman, K. (2022). Veterinary house officer perceptions of dimensions of well-being during postgraduate training. *Journal of the American Veterinary Medical Association* 260 (11): 1369–1376.

Merck Animal Health (2023). *Veterinary Wellbeing Study: Improving Wellbeing and Mental Health, 2024*. Merck &

Co., Inc. https://www.merck-animal-health-usa.com/offload-downloads/2023-vet-wellbeing-presentation (accessed 17 March 2024).

Morello, S. (2023). Resident and intern salaries: can tracking our progress help us understand our future? *Journal of the American Veterinary Medical Association* 261 (5): 758–765.

Morello, S., Shiu, K., and Thurston, J. (2021). Comparison of resident and intern salaries with the current living wage as a quantitative estimate of financial strain among post-graduate veterinary trainees. *Journal of the American Veterinary Medical Association* 260 (1): 124–132.

Mulligan, E.P., Dickson, T., and DeVahl, J. (2020). Financial literacy among health professions graduate students. *Journal of Allied Health 49* (3): 181–189.

National Association of Veterinary Technicians in America (NAVTA) (2022). *Demographic Survey Results: Pay & Education Have Increased; Burnout & Debt Are Still Issues.* National Association of Veterinary Technicians in America. https://drive.google.com/file/d/11pmYzIouybfL55YsduRbaZ1TtMD1i2DB/view (accessed 23 March 2024).

National Association of Veterinary Technicians in America (NAVTA) (2024). NAVTA demographic survey results 2024: title protection, income, role clarity, and wellness within the veterinary technician profession. Bridgewater, NJ: NAVTA.

NerdWallet. (2024). Compound Interest Calculator. *NerdWallet.* Available at: https://www.nerdwallet.com/banking/calculators/compound-interest-calculator Opens a new window (accessed: 20 April 2026).

Reinhard, A.R., Celt, V.P., Pilewki, L.E., and Hendricks, M.K. (2025). The newly credentialed veterinary technician: perceptions, realities, and career challenges. *Frontiers in Veterinary Science 12*: 1437525.

Roasa, L. (2022). What is happening with bonuses in veterinary practice? *VIN News Service.* https://news.vin.com/default.aspx?pid=210&Id=10912435&f5=1 (accessed 14 September 2024).

Scoresby, K., Jurney, C., Fackler, A. et al. (2023). Relationships between diversity demographics, psychological distress, and suicidal thinking in the veterinary profession: a nationwide cross-sectional study during COVID-19. *Frontiers in Veterinary Science 10*: 1130826.

Silverman, E. (2016). Female veterinarians can expect less pay — and that's baked into this salary calculator. *STAT*, 25 May. Available at: STAT website (accessed 20 April 2026).

Singler, E. New legislation limits federal student loan options for veterinary students. *AAHA Trends.* https://www.aaha.org/trends-magazine/publications/new-legislation-limits-federal-student-loan-options-for-veterinary-students/ (accessed 30 October 2025).

Steffey, M.A., Griffon, D.J., Risselada, M. et al. (2023). A narrative review of the physiology and health effects of burnout associated with veterinarian-pertinent occupational stressors. *Frontiers in Veterinary Science 10*: 1184525.

U.S. Bureau of Labor Statistics (2025). *Veterinary Technologists and Technicians.* Occupational Outlook Handbook. https://www.bls.gov/ooh/healthcare/veterinary-technologists-and-technicians.htm (accessed 14 December 2025).

Volk, J.O., Schimmack, U., Strand, E.B. et al. (2018). Executive summary of the Merck animal health veterinary wellbeing study. *Journal of the American Veterinary Medical Association* 252 (10): 1231–1238.

Volk, J.O., Schimmack, U., Strand, E.B. et al. (2024). Merck Animal Health Veterinary Team study reveals factors associated with well-being, burnout, and mental health among nonveterinarian practice team members. *Journal of the American Veterinary Medical Association* 262 (10): 1330–1337.

Volk, J.O., Schimmack, U., Strand, E.B. et al. (2022). Executive summary of the Merck Animal Health Veterinarian Wellbeing Study III and Veterinary Support Staff Study. *Journal of the American Veterinary Medical Association* 260 (12): 1547–1553.

Volk, J.O., Schimmack, U., Strand, E.B. et al. (2020). Executive summary of the Merck animal health veterinarian wellbeing study II. *Journal of the American Veterinary Medical Association* 256 (11): 1237–1244.

Warren, E. and Tyagi, A. (2005). *All Your Worth: The Ultimate Lifetime Money Plan*, 26.

Zakharenkov, I. (2023). Does production pay undermine veterinary team well-being? *VIN News Service.* https://news.vin.com/default.aspx?pid=210&Id=11545511&f5=1 (accessed Jul 28, 2024).

Zoetis, (2024). Veterinarian production pay versus salary: how does it work?. *Zoetis Petcare*, 14 October. Available at: https://www.zoetisus.com/petcare/blog/veterinarian-production-pay-versus-salary (accessed 20 April 2026).National Association of Veterinary Technicians in America (NAVTA) (2024). NAVTA demographic survey results 2024: title protection, income, role clarity, and wellness within the veterinary technician profession. Bridgewater, NJ: NAVTA.

Burnout

CHAPTER 9

Carrie Jurney, DVM, DACVIM (Neurology)[1], Malissa Clark, PhD[2], and Skylar Oney, MS[2]

[1] *Not One More Vet, Inc, San Francisco, CA, USA*

[2] *Department of Pyschology, University of Georgia, Athens, GA, USA*

INTRODUCTION

Burnout is often described as exhaustion or stress from work-related problems, but exhaustion alone does not encompass the full experience of burnout. Burnout also brings a sense of cynicism, detachment, and/or disengagement from work tasks. People experiencing burnout mentally distance themselves from their work and have an inability and/or unwillingness to engage fully with the tasks assigned to them. Finally, decline in work performance may occur in addition to or as a consequence of exhaustion and detachment (Desart and De Witte 2019; Maslach 1976). With further study, researchers have included other cognitive, psychological, and physical consequences of burnout, which this chapter discusses in depth. All in all, the definition of burnout paints a picture of a person who is not only physically and emotionally drained but also mentally strained, struggling to cope with the demands of their work and daily life.

Interestingly, the earliest explorations of burnout were focused on healthcare professionals and other individuals who did a lot of "people work" (Maslach 1976). It's therefore no surprise that burnout is prevalent among veterinary professionals. Research of various veterinary populations has shown burnout rates ranging from about one-third to over half of those examined (Kogan et al. 2020; Ouedraogo et al. 2021; Steffey et al. 2023; Volk et al. 2022). These figures parallel or surpass the rates observed in equivalent roles in human healthcare and exceed those found in the general population (Ouedraogo et al. 2021; Volk et al. 2020). In this chapter, we will explore the effects of burnout, as well as risk factors, prevention strategies, and recovery.

THE EFFECTS OF BURNOUT

Burnout is defined as an occupational phenomenon rather than a specific medical condition (WHO Departmental Update 2019). While it may not be classified alone as a medical condition, burnout has been associated with various emotional, physical, and cognitive consequences that warrant examination.

The emotional repercussions of burnout are typically the most apparent, as burnout is commonly defined by its impact on mental and emotional well-being (e.g. exhaustion, cynicism, disengagement). Aside from these emotional experiences, studies have linked burnout to defined mental health conditions such as depression, suicidal ideation, and anxiety (Nadon et al. 2022). The correlation with depression is particularly strong in the general population, and was also found in a study of veterinary technicians in four specialty hospitals (Hayes et al. 2020; Nadon et al. 2022). Burnout and depression share many symptoms like helplessness, hopelessness, negative affect, and difficulty feeling positive emotions. However, they are most consistently considered separate conditions with reciprocal associations (Nadon et al. 2022). In veterinarians, burnout was also found to mediate the impact of workplace stressors on suicidal ideation (Andela 2021). Given the concern for increased rates of suicidality in veterinarians, this highlights the need for both burnout prevention and treatment.

Burnout can also impact our cognitive capabilities. In a meta-analysis spanning 17 studies, burnout was associated with impaired memory, executive functioning, attention, and processing speed (Gavelin et al. 2022). In a fast-paced environment, where functional memory of multiple patients as well as recall of a large volume of medical information is required to perform the tasks of the job, it's easy to see how burnout could impact job performance. Unsurprisingly, in another large meta-analysis looking at over 20,000 physicians, there was a 2.72-fold increase in self-reported errors in clinicians experiencing burnout (Owoc et al. 2022). Similar increased error rates have been reported in veterinary technicians (Hayes et al. 2020). Burnout and medical errors may also become part of a vicious cycle, as physicians experiencing burnout are more likely to report medical errors, and those reporting medical errors are more likely to consequently experience burnout (Steffey et al. 2023). Other aspects of care (e.g. communication, use of best practices, patient outcomes) may also be impacted by burnout. However, these associations are not as consistently supported in the literature as burnout's impact on medical errors (Tawfik et al. 2019). Ultimately, consequences of burnout, namely turnover and reduction of hours, have been estimated to cost the US veterinary industry 2 billion dollars annually in lost revenue (Neill et al. 2022).

The consequences of burnout do not end with its emotional and cognitive impacts. Burnout has also appeared to have a reciprocal relationship with various physical health conditions (von Känel et al. 2020). For instance, social workers experiencing burnout have higher levels of physical health conditions, leading to faster physical health deterioration over one year (Kim et al. 2011). The different aspects of burnout are also associated with certain somatic diseases. For instance, people with higher levels of exhaustion have a 40% increased risk of high blood pressure, while those with lower levels of personal efficacy have a 47% increase in risk of chronic lung diseases (von Känel et al. 2020). Overall, a single-point increase on the Maslach Burnout Inventory has been associated with a 35% increase in all-cause mortality (Ahola et al. 2010). See Table 9.1 for a list of chronic health conditions associated with burnout.

Table 9.1 Somatic conditions directly associated with burnout in peer-reviewed literature.

Somatic condition	Evidence summary
Musculoskeletal pain (e.g. back, neck)	Burnout predicts musculoskeletal pain and changes in pain perception over time (Salvagioni et al. 2017; Edú-Valsania et al. 2022)
Headaches	Increased prevalence of headaches observed among individuals with burnout (Salvagioni et al. 2017)
Gastrointestinal issues	Prospective studies report higher rates of gastric disturbances and bowel irritation in burnout (Salvagioni et al. 2017; Edú-Valsania et al. 2022)
Sleep disturbances/ insomnia	Strongly associated; burnout is linked with insomnia and impaired sleep quality (Salvagioni et al. 2017; Edú-Valsania et al. 2022)
Type 2 diabetes	Longitudinal studies show burnout increases risk of type 2 diabetes (Salvagioni et al. 2017)
Hypercholesterolemia	Burnout predicts development of hypercholesterolemia (Salvagioni et al. 2017)
Coronary heart disease	Burnout prospectively linked to coronary heart disease and cardiovascular morbidity (Salvagioni et al. 2017; von Känel et al. 2020)
High blood pressure	Burnout associated with elevated blood pressure, independent of depression (von Känel et al. 2020)
Chronic lung disease	Low professional efficacy dimension associated with chronic lung disease (von Känel et al. 2020)
Increased inflammatory biomarkers	Burnout associated with dysregulated immune/endocrine activity and elevated pro-inflammatory markers (Toker et al. 2012)

BURNOUT RISK FACTORS AND THEIR PREVENTION

Within veterinary medicine, different roles and aspects are associated with different levels of burnout. For instance, veterinarians who spend over 75% of their practice on small animal medicine have higher burnout levels than those who do not (Ouedraogo et al. 2021). In 2023, the Pew Research Center reported that over half of Americans now consider their pets as important in their family as human family members (Brown 2023). Practitioners treating these animals are therefore faced with heightened expectations accompanied by increased levels of conflict, moral dilemmas, and fears of professional mistakes, which can set the stage for burnout (Ouedraogo et al. 2021). Academic veterinarians also have elevated burnout rates compared to their private practice peers, which is reportedly due to work overload and a lack of autonomy to make changes within their workplaces (Adin et al. 2023). House officers report elevated levels of burnout, likely secondary to increased job demands and a lack of personal resources (Chigerwe et al. 2021). Conversely, private practice owners tend to experience lower burnout levels, largely attributed to the autonomy they wield in managing their practices, alongside higher earning potential (Ouedraogo et al. 2021). Importantly, these studies cannot establish causal linkages between the area of veterinary medicine we choose (i.e. academic vs private, small animal vs large animal) or our role in that community (e.g. house officer and practice owner) and burnout, but this research can shed light on different sets of challenges and stressors in our environments that may contribute to burnout. Thankfully, protective measures can be taken to mitigate these challenges.

The Job Demands-Resources Model (JD-R) was first utilized to explain the interplay among the variety of tasks we are asked to do in our work, the tools we are given to accomplish them, and how a mismatch of the two can result in burnout (Demerouti et al. 2001). Figure 9.1 describes the interaction of demands and resources with exhaustion and engagement at work (Mastenbroek 2017). As shown in this figure, both individual and organizational elements mediate engagement and exhaustion. In an analysis of both veterinarians and technicians in Australia, organizational and individual factors both contributed to variance in burnout scores to a similar degree (47.9% and 45.3%, respectively). However, other studies show that organizational factors have a greater degree of influence than individual factors (Rohlf et al. 2022; Lesener et al. 2020).

Overall, both organizational and individual factors play a role in our experience of burnout and/or engagement and are worthy of attention. Many of these concepts have been discussed at length in Chapters 2, 6, and 7. However, several studies have directly related certain organizational and individual factors to burnout within veterinary populations.

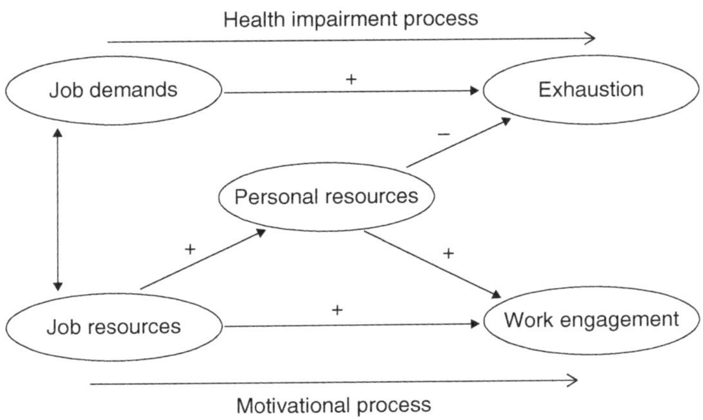

FIGURE 9.1 Jobs Demands-Resources Model. Mastenbroek et al. (2014) / John Wiley & Sons.

ORGANIZATIONAL FACTORS

The impact organizations can have on well-being was covered in depth in Chapter 7, and unsurprisingly, organizational factors also impact burnout. In a study of veterinary technicians, two strong themes emerged as organizational risk factors for burnout: conflict and workload (Hayes et al. 2020).

As discussed in Chapter 6, conflict is common in veterinary medicine, and all forms of conflict (e.g. supervisor, client, and colleague) have been shown to increase burnout in veterinary professionals (Ashton-James and McNeilage 2022; Hayes et al. 2020; Irwin et al. 2022). Alternatively, positive workplace culture (e.g. feeling respected and good social support from colleagues) is protective within the veterinary community (Kogan et al. 2020; Liss et al. 2020; Rohlf et al. 2022). Organizations that foster communicative and respectful workplaces are therefore less likely to contribute to burnout. Cultivating a positive work environment may also help address the burnout risk from work overload, as human nurses who reported factors such as "workplace commitment," "a cohesive team," and "recognition from supervisors" showed weaker associations between workload and burnout than their counterparts without these resources (Diehl et al. 2021). Chapter 7 discusses the ingredients of a healthy workplace culture and the importance of well-being in detail.

Workload was identified as the top stressor in a study of veterinary professionals, 58% of whom were experiencing burnout (Ashton-James and McNeilage 2022). Multiple studies have echoed this finding – our workloads are a primary driver of negative well-being, specifically burnout (Adin et al. 2023; Ashton-James and McNeilage 2022; Hayes et al. 2020). Work overload can be related to a variety of clinical factors, such as staffing, patient volume, time allotted per patient, and available administrative time; all of which are opportunities for organizational prevention of burnout (Steffey et al. 2023). Within human medicine, a 10% decrease in responsibilities for physicians resulted in a 33% reduction in burnout risk (Harry et al. 2021).

Another key protective theme for veterinary professionals is personal development. The ability to learn, be coached on, and use new skills is protective against burnout in both veterinarians and technicians (Kogan et al. 2020; Mastenbroek et al. 2014). While the drive to seek continuing education and personal development is up to the individual, it is often impacted by organizational factors such as the availability of skilled mentors, continuing education (CE) funding, and time off to pursue educational opportunities.

INDIVIDUAL FACTORS

Individual factors account for 45% of the variance in burnout in veterinary professionals (Rohlf et al. 2022). Demographically speaking, both age and gender have been found to relate to burnout. Additionally, personality traits, as well as mental skill sets, can have an impact on the experience of burnout.

As age increases, well-being typically improves, and burnout is no exception (Volk et al. 2022; Ouedraogo et al. 2021). In fact, years since graduation was the single strongest protection against burnout in one study of veterinarians (Ouedraogo et al. 2021). However, it may not be age itself, but rather experience, driving this effect. In a study of Canadian veterinarians, when controlling for other factors, there was no correlation between age and burnout or other mental health metrics (Perret et al. 2020). The impact of experience suggests that we acquire skills over time, which lessen the impact of stressors, or that, with time, we may gain more autonomy within our profession, providing protection against burnout. It is also possible that as one acquires greater levels of skill and experience, one is able to accomplish a similar workload more efficiently. However, it may also be related to survivor bias in that over time, burned-out individuals may leave the profession and no longer be included in sample populations (Ouedraogo et al. 2021).

Gender presents a similarly complicated picture. Across multiple well-being and mental health metrics, women tend to fare worse than men (Ouedraogo et al. 2021; Volk et al. 2022; Mastenbroek et al. 2014; Kogan et al. 2020). However, once again, caution should be taken in mistaking cause and effect. Rather than gender itself being causally implicated, gender-based differences in workplace stressors may contribute to the higher levels of burnout reported among women (Steffey et al. 2023). For example, workplace gender discrimination is the most frequent form of discrimination in veterinary medicine (Summers et al. 2023). Additionally, there may be confounding variables unaccounted for across studies. For instance, female veterinary professionals have been found to have higher levels of empathy, and while this is a necessary trait in medicine, it is also a risk factor for the emotional exhaustion aspect of burnout (Colombo et al. 2017; Varela and Correia 2023). There could also be psychosocial factors at play, as women tend to be more willing to disclose distress, which is evidenced by lower self-stigma toward mental health care in female veterinary students (Knight et al. 2019; Qiu et al. 2024).

Other personality factors have also been linked to burnout. When faced with a challenging circumstance, veterinary professionals who tend to disengage or self-blame have higher levels of burnout (Rohlf et al. 2022). Conversely, individuals with higher levels of optimism, emotional intelligence, and self-compassion tend to have lower levels of burnout (Rohlf et al. 2022). As discussed in Chapter 2, while most personality traits are at least partially genetic, they also involve aspects of experience and training. If individuals do not naturally tend toward these protective traits, they are, at least in part, a teachable skill. These skills will be discussed in depth in Chapter 10.

Having children and spending time with family are both associated with decreased burnout among veterinary professionals (Ouedraogo et al. 2021; Volk et al. 2022). However, broader work–family studies offer a more nuanced picture: having children is associated with lower burnout. Still, when children are young and family time is primarily spent on household chores, burnout is higher (ten Brummelhuis et al. 2008). Finding a balance between work and home life is particularly important for veterinary professionals. Many individuals in the field consider the work a calling, and 41% of veterinary students say they have wanted to be a veterinarian as long as they can remember (Moody 2022; Strand et al. 2017). This calling can be protective against burnout (Moody 2022). However, when paired with certain traits like perfectionism, a strong sense of professional identity becomes a risk factor for burnout in veterinary professionals (Moody 2022; Varela and Correia 2023).

FINANCES AND BURNOUT

Financial matters walk the line between organizational and personal issues. The particulars of a person's debt load or salary vary from person to person, but low income and student debt are identified as profession-wide risk factors for well-being problems (Liss et al. 2020; Volk et al. 2022). In fact, student debt has consistently ranked second among risk factors for negative well-being in veterinarians (Volk et al. 2018, 2020). Interestingly, regardless of the amount of debt, veterinarians who engaged a financial planner not only paid off their debt faster but also had significantly lower distress levels (Volk et al. 2020).

Salary also has an impact on burnout. A 2020 study of veterinary technicians showed that a wage higher than $21.00/hour was associated with higher engagement scores (i.e. the opposite of burnout). Similarly, higher incomes are protective against burnout in veterinarians (Ouedraogo et al. 2021). Interestingly, while higher salaries correlate with lower burnout rates, common compensation strategies such as production-based pay may inadvertently contribute to burnout (Steffey et al. 2023). This association has been observed in physicians, where production-based compensation was linked to a 37% increase in burnout risk (Shanafelt et al. 2009). Multiple factors within production-based pay may be behind this risk, including reduced time per patient and moral injury arising from the conflict between patient needs and business-driven healthcare objectives (Steffey et al. 2023).

A full discussion of finances and their impact on well-being is in Chapter 8.

WARNING SIGNS FOR BURNOUT

Most research focuses on the symptoms of established burnout, such as emotional exhaustion, depersonalization, and reduced professional efficacy. However, growing evidence suggests that certain early indicators appear before the full syndrome develops. Recognizing these warning signs allows for earlier intervention and prevention.

Emotional and cognitive changes are often among the first indicators. Reduced enthusiasm, increased irritability, or a growing sense of inefficacy despite stable workloads can all be signs of impending burnout (Steffey et al. 2023). Subtle cognitive shifts, such as diminished concentration or forgetfulness, can also signal burnout (Nagle et al. 2024). In veterinary professionals, periods of heightened moral distress can precede burnout (Kogan et al. 2020).

Behavioral patterns also shift before full burnout. Overcommitment, working longer hours, and a gradual withdrawal from colleagues or team discussions are commonly observed (Steffey et al. 2023). Longitudinal studies in healthcare workers have shown that persistent workload increases burnout without adequate rest, and declining social connection often precedes burnout (Salvagioni et al. 2017).

Physiological changes can provide additional early signals. Sleep disruption, fatigue, and tension, such as musculoskeletal pain or headaches, may reflect chronic activation of the stress response (Toker et al. 2012; von Känel et al. 2020). These signs are frequently misinterpreted as normal occupational fatigue, which can delay recognition. There is a difference between feeling tired after a long, productive day and feeling chronic fatigue and exhaustion that may be a sign of burnout.

In summary, early warning signs of burnout often include declining motivation, cognitive fog, irritability, sleep problems, fatigue, and physical discomfort. Detecting and addressing these signals early through rest, reflection, and supportive relationships may prevent progression to full burnout.

RECOVERY FROM BURNOUT

Although much is known about burnout itself, understanding its recovery process is still a work in progress. Research shows that employees who continue engaging in work-related activities during off-job time experience lower daily recovery (i.e. day-to-day recovery experiences, compared to more permanent, long-term recovery); yet, engaging in nonwork activities is quite effective in facilitating burnout recovery (Oerlemans and Bakker 2014). Preventative factors, such as engaging in social (e.g. time with friends and family) and low-effort (e.g. relaxing or resting) activities, are particularly helpful in facilitating higher recovery, especially for employees at greater risk of burnout (Oerlemans and Bakker 2014). Given these findings, it's no surprise that spending time with family and friends has been associated with lower burnout in veterinary populations (Ouedraogo et al. 2021).

Limited research in healthcare residency programs has revealed that some of the highest-impact burnout recovery factors include changing rotations, increased sleep, and meaningful colleague relationships (Tang et al. 2020). Efforts by employers to facilitate outdoor activities and social events across programs also proved helpful in resident recovery (Tang et al. 2020). Additionally, as jobs become more stressful, stable support resources (e.g. healthy leadership and human resources practices) become increasingly important in employee regulation of short-term fatigue and avoiding long-term burnout (Bakker and de Vries 2021). Perhaps the most focal areas to consider for the workplace are increasing variety in job rotations, fostering valuable social interactions and relationships, reducing workload, and ensuring stable support resources are available.

Aside from the above, knowledge of how to effectively treat burnout is lacking in both research and practice. Most known interventions are prevention-focused and have small positive effects but do not significantly impact employees already suffering from burnout (Demerouti et al. 2021). While various research teams are working to identify effective strategies to reduce the psychological symptoms of burnout and effectively reintegrate burned-out employees, little conclusive evidence exists. Thus far, it is only clear that burnout recovery is two-pronged and will rely on both job redesign and symptom treatment to effectively combat burnout's primary drivers (van Dam 2021). Story 9.1 provides two stories of burnout, one from a technician and another from a veterinarian. In both instances, a period of rest and a new role were a part of their recovery.

STORY 9.1 A VETERINARIAN'S EXPERIENCE WITH BURNOUT

I had finished school and started my first real job. I had no life. I was so used to school being everything. Now I had some free time, and I didn't know what to do with it. So naturally I went to work. There was always some case that needed me, a record to write, a phone call to make, so it was an easy excuse. And as I started to burn out, I mistakenly concluded it was due to my lack of control and management's actions. So I started a practice with some friends, and boy, was that stupid. I, a person with no boundaries who was already burnt out, took on a herculean task. Starting a practice is all-consuming; it pulls you in a million directions, and you have to learn a lot very quickly. And after two years of that, I broke. I quit my job. I don't think I moved from my couch for two weeks. Then I started taking walks, hanging out with friends, and slowly started to remember who I was. I was scared to return to clinical practice, so I started looking at jobs in industry, research, and government. After a few months of surfing job ads, I couldn't find anything that felt like a good fit. I decided to come back to clinical medicine, but I did it very differently. I didn't want to commit to full-time practice again, so I started to work as a relief doctor. This gave me firm boundaries on schedule. I was often covering clinics in other states, so there was no way I could pop in on my day off. Because of the nature of my contracts, I had to pass the cases off to the doctors who worked there full time, so there was no follow-up to do. I also started to work hard on all of those other parts of my life that I had neglected for too long: my hobbies, volunteering, my family. Low and behold it worked. I wasn't burned out anymore. Much to my chagrin I was doing a much better job, making just as much money, working two weeks a month as I did working full-time, 60-hour weeks. After a couple of years, I returned to full-time practice, and in the last year I've started another practice. It's going much better this time. Now, I keep a close eye on my boundaries and any feelings of burnout. Prevention is way, way better than the painful process of recovery.

A Technician's Experience with Burnout:

I was burned out working graveyard shift in the ER during crazy COVID times. We wouldn't turn anyone away even though we all had way more patients than we could handle in the ICU. I was always hours behind on treatments and felt like I was failing my patients. The last straw was when I was concerned about a patient and the doctor wouldn't come look at it. I tried to get her several times throughout the night. It wasn't until 20 minutes before my shift ended, when the pet coded, did she come. The dog died in my arms and I was PISSED! I left that job, did a short stint out of the field (nine months) and still picked up a few relief shifts. I stopped vet med entirely from mid-February to June when I started looking for another vet ER job. Now I'm at a new location, working days, and all good. December will be 20 years in the field for me.

REFERENCES

Adin, C.A., Stefanou, C.R., and Merlo, L.J. (2023). Assessment of burnout, professional fulfillment, and strategies for improvement in veterinary faculty at a large academic department. *Journal of Veterinary Medical Education* 50 (1): 53–60.

Ahola, K., Väänänen, A., Koskinen, A. et al. (2010). Burnout as a predictor of all-cause mortality among industrial employees: a 10-year prospective register-linkage study. *Journal of Psychosomatic Research* 69 (1): 51–57.

Andela, M. (2021). Work-related stressors and suicidal ideation: the mediating role of burnout. *Journal of Workplace Behavioral Health* 36 (2): 125–145.

Ashton-James, C.E. and McNeilage, A.G. (2022). A mixed methods investigation of stress and well-being factors contributing to burnout and job satisfaction in a specialist small animal hospital. *Frontiers in Veterinary Science* 9: 942778.

Bakker, A.B. and de Vries, J.D. (2021). Job Demands–Resources theory and self-regulation: new explanations and remedies for job burnout. *Anxiety, Stress, and Coping* 34 (1): 1–21.

Brown, A. (2023). About half of US pet owners say their pets are as much a part of their family as a human member. *Pew Research Center* 7.

Chigerwe, M., Barter, L., Dechant, J.E. et al. (2021). A preliminary study on assessment of wellbeing among veterinary medical house officers. *PLoS One* 16 (6): e0253111.

Colombo, E.S., Crippa, F., Calderari, T., and Prato-Previde, E. (2017). Empathy toward animals and people: the role of gender and length of service in a sample of Italian veterinarians. *Journal of Veterinary Behavior* 17: 32–37.

Demerouti, E., Bakker, A.B., Nachreiner, F., and Schaufeli, W.B. (2001). The job demands-resources model of burnout. *Journal of Applied Psychology* 86 (3): 499.

Demerouti, E., Bakker, A.B., Peeters, M.C.W., and Breevaart, K. (2021). New directions in burnout research. *European Journal of Work and Organizational Psychology* 30 (5): 686–691. https://doi.org/10.1080/1359432X.2021.1979962.

Desart, S. and De Witte, H. (2019). Burnout 2.0 – a new look at the conceptualization of burn-out. In: *The Fun and Frustration of Modern Working Life* (ed. T. Taris, M. Peeters, and H. De Witte), 1430–1152. Kalmthout: Pelckmans Pro.

Diehl, E., Rieger, S., Letzel, S. et al. (2021). The relationship between workload and burnout among nurses: the buffering role of personal, social and organizational resources. *PLoS One* 16 (1): e0245798.

Edú-Valsania, S., Laguía, A., and Moriano, J.A. (2022). Burnout: A review of theory and measurement. *International Journal of Environmental Research and Public Health* 19 (3): 1780.

Gavelin, H.M., Domellöf, M.E., Åström, E. et al. (2022). Cognitive function in clinical burnout: a systematic review and meta-analysis. *Work & Stress* 36 (1): 86–104.

Harry, E., Sinsky, C., Dyrbye, L.N. et al. (2021). Physician task load and the risk of burnout among US physicians in a national survey. *The Joint Commission Journal on Quality and Patient Safety* 47 (2): 76–85.

Hayes, G.M., LaLonde-Paul, D.F., Perret, J.L. et al. (2020). Investigation of burnout syndrome and job-related risk factors in veterinary technicians in specialty teaching hospitals: a multicenter cross-sectional study. *Journal of Veterinary Emergency and Critical Care* 30 (1): 18–27.

Irwin, A., Silver-MacMahon, H., and Wilcke, S. (2022). Consequences and coping: investigating client, co-worker and senior colleague incivility within veterinary practice. *Veterinary Record* 191 (7).

Kim, H., Ji, J., and Kao, D. (2011). Burnout and physical health among social workers: a three-year longitudinal study. *Social Work* 258–268.

Knight, M.L. et al. (2019). Cross-sectional analysis of veterinary student coping strategies and stigma in seeking psychological help. *Veterinary Record* 184 (23): 709.

Kogan, L.R., Wallace, J.E., Schoenfeld-Tacher, R. et al. (2020). Veterinary technicians and occupational burnout. *Frontiers in Veterinary Science* 7: 328.

Lesener, T., Gusy, B., Jochmann, A., and Wolter, C. (2020). The drivers of work engagement: a meta-analytic review of longitudinal evidence. *Work & Stress* 34 (3): 259–278.

Liss, D.J., Kerl, M.E., and Tsai, C.L. (2020). Factors associated with job satisfaction and engagement among credentialed small animal veterinary technicians in the United States. *Journal of the American Veterinary Medical Association* 257 (5): 537–545.

Maslach, C. (1976). Burned-out. *Human Behavior* 5: 16–22.

Mastenbroek, N.J. (2017). The art of staying engaged: the role of personal resources in the mental well-being of young veterinary professionals. *Journal of Veterinary Medical Education* 44 (1): 84–94.

Mastenbroek, N.J.J.M., Jaarsma, A.D.C., Demerouti, E. et al. (2014). Burnout and engagement, and its predictors in young veterinary professionals: the influence of gender. *Veterinary Record* 174 (6): 144.

Ciobanu, A.M., Damian, A.C., and Neagu, C. (2021). Association between burnout and immunological and endocrine alterations. *Romanian Journal of Morphology and Embryology* 62 (1): 13.

Moody, A.B. (2022). The dark side of calling: a partial test of the work as calling theory (WCT) using the veterinarian occupational well-being study (VOWS). Doctoral dissertation. Colorado State University.

Nadon, L., De Beer, L.T., and Morin, A.J. (2022). Should burnout be conceptualized as a mental disorder? *Behavioral Science* 12 (3): 82.

Nagle, E., Griskevica, I., Rajevska, O. et al. (2024). Factors affecting healthcare workers burnout and their conceptual models: scoping review. *BMC Psychology* 12 (1): 637.

Neill, C.L., Hansen, C.R., and Salois, M. (2022). The economic cost of burnout in veterinary medicine. *Frontiers in Veterinary Science* 9: 814104.

Oerlemans, W.G.M. and Bakker, A.B. (2014). Burnout and daily recovery: a day reconstruction study. *Journal of Occupational Health Psychology* 19 (3): 303–314. https://doi.org/10.1037/a0036904.

Ouedraogo, F.B., Lefebvre, S.L., Hansen, C.R., and Wade Brorsen, B. (2021). Compassion satisfaction, burnout, and secondary traumatic stress among full-time veterinarians in the United States (2016–2018). *Journal of the American Veterinary Medical Association* 258 (11): 1259–1270.

Owoc, J., Mańczak, M., Jabłońska, M. et al. (2022). Association between physician burnout and self-reported errors: meta-analysis. *Journal of Patient Safety* 18 (1): e180–e188.

Perret, J.L., Best, C.O., Coe, J.B. et al. (2020). Association of demographic, career, and lifestyle factors with resilience and association of resilience with mental health outcomes in veterinarians in Canada. *Journal of the American Veterinary Medical Association* 257: 1057–1068.

Qiu, L., Xu, H., Li, Y. et al. (2024). Gender differences in attitudes towards psychological help: women tend to be more willing to disclose their emotions than men. *BMC Public Health*.

Rohlf, V.I., Scotney, R., Monaghan, H., and Bennett, P. (2022). Predictors of professional quality of life in veterinary professionals. *Journal of Veterinary Medical Education* 49 (3): 372–381.

Salvagioni, D.A.J., Melanda, F.N., Mesas, A.E. et al. (2017). Physical, psychological and occupational consequences of job burnout: A systematic review of prospective studies. *PLoS One* 12 (10): e0185781.

Shanafelt, T.D., Balch, C.M., Bechamps, G.J. et al. (2009). Burnout and career satisfaction among American surgeons. *Annals of Surgery* 250 (3): 463–471.

Steffey, M.A., Griffon, D.J., Risselada, M. et al. (2023). Veterinarian burnout demographics and organizational impacts: a narrative review. *Frontiers in Veterinary Science* 10: 1184526.

Strand, E.B., Brandt, J., Rogers, K. et al. (2017). Adverse childhood experiences among veterinary medical students: a multi-site study. *Journal of Veterinary Medical Education* 44 (2): 260–267.

Summers, O.S., Medcalf, R., Hubbard, K.A., and McCarroll, C.S. (2023). A cross-sectional study examining perceptions of discriminatory behaviors experienced and witnessed by veterinary students undertaking clinical extra-mural studies. *Frontiers in Veterinary Science* 10: 940836.

Tang, O.Y., Dunn, K.A., Yoon, J.S. et al. (2020). Neurosurgery resident wellness and recovery from burnout: a 39-year single-institution experience. *World Neurosurgery* 138: https://doi.org/10.1016/j.wneu.2020.01.236.

Tawfik, D.S., Scheid, A., Profit, J. et al. (2019). Evidence relating health care provider burnout and quality of care: a systematic review and meta-analysis. *Annals of Internal Medicine* 171 (8): 555–567.

ten Brummelhuis, L., van der Lippe, T., Kluwer, E.S., and Flap, H. (2008). Positive and negative effects of family involvement on work-related burnout. *Journal of Vocational Behavior* 73: 387–396.

Toker, S., Shirom, A., Shapira, I. et al. (2012). Burnout and serum levels of inflammation markers: a longitudinal study. *Psychoneuroendocrinology* 37 (5): 742–752.

van Dam, A. (2021). A clinical perspective on burnout: diagnosis, classification, and treatment of clinical burnout. *European Journal of Work and Organizational Psychology* 30 (5): 732–741. https://doi.org/10.1080/1359432X.2021.1948400.

Varela, M. and Correia, I. (2023). Empathy and burnout in veterinarians and veterinary nurses: identifying burnout protectors. *Anthrozoös* 36 (1): 15–34.

Volk, J.O., Schimmack, U., Strand, E.B. et al. (2018). Executive summary of the Merck animal health veterinary wellbeing study. *Journal of the American Veterinary Medical Association* 252 (10): 1231–1238.

Volk, J.O., Schimmack, U., Strand, E.B. et al. (2022). Executive summary of the Merck Animal Health

Veterinarian Wellbeing Study III and Veterinary Support Staff Study. *Journal of the American Veterinary Medical Association* 260 (12): 1547–1553.

Volk, J.O., Schimmack, U., Strand, E.B. et al. (2020). Executive summary of the Merck animal health veterinarian wellbeing study II. *Journal of the American Veterinary Medical Association* 256 (11): 1237–1244.

von Känel, R., Princip, M., Holzgang, S.A. et al. (2020). Relationship between job burnout and somatic diseases: a network analysis. *Scientific Reports* 10 (1): 18438.

World Health Organization, Departmental Update (2019). Burn-out an 'Occupational phenomenon': International Classification of Diseases, World Health Organization. https://www.who.int/news/item/28-05-2019-burn-out-an-occupational-phenomenon-international-classification-of-diseases (accessed 23 September 2024).

Positive Psychology

CHAPTER 10

Carrie Jurney, DVM, DACVIM (Neurology)[1],
Olivia Knizek, PhD, CMPC[2], and Zachary Ward, PhD[3]

[1] *Not One More Vet, Inc, San Francisco, CA, USA*
[2] *Student Health & Counseling Services, University of California Davis, Davis, CA, USA*
[3] *School of Veterinary Medicine, University of California Davis, Davis, CA, USA*

INTRODUCTION

In the first chapter of this book, we highlighted the importance of positive action for well-being, accounting for approximately 40% of our happiness (Lyubomirsky et al. 2005). Positive psychology is the branch of science that studies how we can improve and maintain our well-being. Throughout this text, we have also discussed positive psychology interventions such as mindfulness and gratitude exercises without spending too much time on their theoretical foundations and empirical evidence. This chapter will seek to remedy that and provide examples of interventions that have been helpful to veterinary professionals.

Scientifically minded individuals are occasionally resistant to these practices, as they are often co-opted by pseudoscientific practitioners. In this context, they may be purported to be a life-changing, cure-all solution for every aspect of life. This understandably can make more scientifically minded individuals doubt their credibility. The reality is that skills like mindfulness will not fix every problem. They will not reverse a surgical error. However, they might help you to process the emotional impact of that difficult situation and reach emotional homeostasis. This homeostasis, in turn, allows you to move on to problem-solving and growth, which in turn are beneficial to subjective well-being (Samsari and Soulis 2019).

Just as these techniques are not necessarily a universal salve for every circumstance, not every tool is right for every situation. Different techniques need to be evaluated on an individual basis and in light of the circumstances for maximal effectiveness (Ciarrochi et al. 2022). Many of these exercises can be practiced on your own. Still, some may find that guidance from a mental health professional is helpful in choosing which exercises will support them in a specific situation. The rest of this chapter will serve as an introduction to a variety of interventions that have been shown to positively impact well-being. This list is by no means exhaustive; rather, it is intended as a jumping-off point for personal exploration of well-being interventions.

HEALTHY COPING

The strategies contained within this chapter help build a physical and mental skillset that allows us not only to feel better in our day-to-day lives but also to cope with stressful situations. Psychologists Lazarus and Folkman (1984) categorized coping into two broad types:

- Problem-focused coping involves directly addressing the source of stress, such as making a plan, solving a problem, or setting a boundary.
- Emotion-focused coping helps regulate the emotional response to a stressor by using strategies such as seeking support, reframing the situation, or practicing acceptance.

At first glance, problem-focused coping may seem superior, and indeed this is supported in the literature (Srivastava et al. 2023). Imagine a veterinarian consistently running late on appointments, frustrating clients, and overwhelming the team. The preferable solution is to analyze and adjust either the schedule or workload to meet the current demands, not to meditate on the stress caused by their lack of punctuality. Yet real-world challenges are rarely this simple. Many stressors in veterinary medicine, such as the exposure to the trauma of others, are inherent to the job and cannot be "solved." These situations call for a blended approach, often relying heavily on emotion-focused strategies. Even when a problem-focused solution exists, emotional coping can help create the mindset needed to act (Srivastava et al. 2023). For instance, after a medical error, self-compassion exercises may be necessary to work through guilt before moving on to corrective steps. Effective coping isn't about choosing one strategy over another. It's about knowing when and how to use both.

Problem-focused coping will be explored further in the section on occupational self-care. Emotion-focused coping strategies, meanwhile, can take many forms: mindfulness, self-compassion, exercise, and social support are all key tools for adaptive coping. Regardless of the methodology, the importance of having healthy coping strategies is clear. The Merck Veterinary Wellbeing Study found that veterinarians with clear coping strategies report higher well-being and lower burnout, with healthy coping mechanisms reported by only 34% of veterinarians with serious psychological distress, compared with 81% of veterinarians who did not report serious distress (Volk et al. 2022). Support staff fared even worse, with lower rates of healthy coping and higher rates of burnout and psychological distress, underscoring the need for intentional strategies across the board (Volk et al. 2022). Building a toolkit of diverse coping skills helps professionals navigate stress more effectively and sustain resilience over the long term. Much of this toolkit involves daily routines and skills that are built in advance of stressful situations, which fall under the umbrella of self-care.

SELF-CARE

What does the phrase "self-care" summon to your imagination? Perhaps it's a bubble bath and bonbons? The World Health Organization defines self-care as "the ability of individuals, families, and communities to promote and maintain their own health, prevent disease, and cope with illness, with or without the support of a health or care worker" (WHO 2024). Unfortunately, chocolate does not seem to be central to their definition. As stated so eloquently by Wiest (2024), "True self-care is not salt baths and chocolate cake; it is making the choice to build a life you don't need to regularly escape from. It means being the hero of your life, not the victim. And that often takes doing the thing you least want to do."

In Chapter 1, we addressed the nuance in the definition of well-being, including the concept of homeostasis. Self-care is part of maintaining our well-being homeostasis, and when done correctly, it is more focused on building healthy habits than indulgences. It's important to acknowledge, as we dive into a discussion of self-care, that it is best achieved through small steps. A large change can be overwhelming and is often unsustainable. However, committing to small steps, like a daily five-minute meditation or setting an alarm to remind yourself to go to bed on time, is much more achievable and sustainable (Gardner et al. 2012).

So what are the components of self-care? Dr. Peggy Swarbrick, Director and Research Professor at Rutgers' Graduate School of Applied and Professional Psychology, first published her eight dimensions of wellness in 1997. That framework has since been widely adopted by organizations such as the Substance Abuse and Mental Health Services Administration in their self-care modules (Swarbrick 1997; SAMHSA 2017). She defines the eight essential aspects of self-care:

1. Emotional: The ability to express emotions, adjust to challenges, and cope with stressful experiences so one can experience joy.
2. Physical: Care of the body, including nutrition, sleep, physical activity, and physical health.
3. Occupational: Engaging in work or volunteer activities that bring satisfaction and enrichment, and also align with personal values and goals.

4. Social: Fostering a sense of belonging and connection in a supportive network of friends, family, and coworkers.
5. Spiritual: Exploring life's purpose and meaning through personal values, religious beliefs, or a sense of connection to something greater than oneself.
6. Intellectual: Engaging in mentally stimulating activities to expand knowledge base and skills.
7. Environmental: Fostering pleasant environments that support well-being.
8. Financial: Attaining a sense of control and satisfaction with your current and future financial situation, ensuring that resources are managed to support a fulfilling and stable life.

This broad model shows that self-care truly isn't restricted to a piece of chocolate cake, nor is a single skill like mindfulness sufficient for a well-rounded self-care strategy. Rather, self-care is a holistic system of caring for many aspects of life. Each of these aspects has an important part to play, and they are also deeply interconnected. For example, a lack of sleep could lead to irritability, which could in turn cause conflict with coworkers in the office. This conflict could then, in turn, cause occupational issues, as well as further sleep problems. Thus, a multifaceted strategy is crucial for success.

It's important to acknowledge that barriers can prevent the implementation of self-care strategies. For instance, feeling overwhelmed or not having the time to implement change is a common barrier to healthy habits (Deslippe et al. 2023). This is ironic, as implementing these habits will help us be more resilient and productive (Grimani et al. 2019; Leipold et al. 2024). This highlights the importance of a growth mindset and deliberate action in self-care.

Some of these aspects of self-care have been addressed in depth in previous chapters. For instance, Chapter 7 focuses on occupational and environmental well-being in the workplace, and Chapter 8 on financial well-being. Similarly, the theme of social self-care, such as work-life balance and nurturing an active social life, has been a consistent theme throughout this text. For the remainder of the chapter, we will focus on the remaining facets of self-care: emotional, physical, occupational, spiritual, and intellectual self-care.

EMOTIONAL SELF-CARE

Emotional self-care is a multidimensional construct, encompassing self-awareness, the regulation and expression of emotions, the cultivation of self-compassion and kindness, the maintenance of boundaries between personal and professional life, and the use of adaptive coping strategies (Dorociak 2015; Keyes et al. 2022). In the following sections, we will cover a few frameworks and coping strategies that have been explicitly examined in veterinary medicine.

EMOTIONAL INTELLIGENCE

Self-awareness, emotional regulation, and expression are central to a skill set known as *emotional intelligence (EQ)*. First described by Thorndike (1920) as social intelligence and later expanded by Salovey and Mayer (1990), EQ is the capacity to understand and manage both one's own emotions and those of others. Rather than a single ability, EQ represents a collection of skills that support coping with stress, particularly in social contexts. Psychologist Travis Bradberry and Greaves (2009) simplifies this framework into four core domains: self-awareness, self-management, social awareness, and relationship management.

Bradberry defines self-awareness as more than simply recognizing one's current emotions; it also involves understanding the values and beliefs that shape them. A critical component of this skill is the ability to identify and articulate emotional states early, creating an opportunity for effective regulation before emotions escalate. This capacity links closely with the practice of mindfulness, which will be discussed later in this section.

In veterinary medicine, higher EQ scores have been associated with lower levels of depression, anxiety, stress, burnout, and secondary traumatic stress, as well as with greater compassion satisfaction among students, house officers, veterinarians, and veterinary support staff (Rohlf et al. 2022; Wells et al. 2021). Yet evidence suggests that veterinary professionals, particularly students and house officers, may begin their training with lower baseline EQ scores compared with other professional groups (Adin et al. 2020). Within these skills, veterinary professionals exhibit strengths such as emotional autonomy and social competencies (e.g. decision-making and social interaction). At the same time, they exhibit relative weaknesses in emotional awareness and regulation (López-López et al. 2025). Encouragingly, training in EQ has been shown to enhance both discrete EQ skills and related well-being outcomes in the general population and among healthcare professionals (Asuero et al. 2014; Hodzic et al. 2018).

For those wishing to deepen their understanding, *Emotional Intelligence: Why It Can Matter More Than IQ* by Daniel Goleman offers an exploration of foundational principles, while *Emotional Intelligence 2.0* by Travis Bradberry and Jean Greaves provides practical strategies for personal growth.

SELF-COMPASSION

> *"There is a certain average tone of self-feeling which each one of us carries about with him, and which is independent of the objective reasons we may have for satisfaction or discontent" (James 1892, pg. 306).*

The Father of American Psychology, William James (1892), offered one of the earliest definitions of self-esteem, describing it as the ratio of our successes to what we believe we are and what we should achieve. More than a century later, Kristin Neff (2003) reframed self-worth through the concept of *self-compassion*, emphasizing self-kindness, common humanity, and mindfulness as pathways to a healthier relationship with oneself. For veterinarians, this perspective is particularly relevant given the profession's strong tendency toward perfectionism (Holden 2020; Karaffa et al. 2024). When perfection becomes the standard, even genuine successes can feel insufficient, undermining self-esteem.

This challenge is evident in the aftermath of professional mistakes. Nearly a quarter of veterinarians report losing confidence in their abilities after an error, even when there are no clinical consequences (Kogan et al. 2018). In Story 10.1, one veterinarian described how a mentor reframed her surgical complication as part of the shared human experience of practicing medicine. This perspective shift enabled her to let go of perfectionist expectations and embrace a more growth-oriented mindset.

Research reflects these lived experiences. Self-compassion is generally lower among veterinary professionals than in the broader population (Hernández-Esteve et al. 2024), yet it is strongly associated with resilience, a greater sense of fulfillment from caregiving work, and lower burnout and secondary traumatic stress (McArthur et al. 2017; Rohlf 2022). Importantly, self-compassion is a trainable skill. Evidence shows that compassion-based interventions can reduce perfectionism, self-criticism, and work-related rumination (Wasson et al. 2020; Wakelin 2021). A pilot study of 128 veterinarians found that an online program significantly improved well-being markers, underscoring the potential of accessible training tools such as those available through Harvard's Stress and Development Lab. Other resources for those interested in working on self-compassion include Dr. Kristin Neff's (2011) Book *Self-Compassion: The Proven Power of Being Kind to Yourself.*

STORY 10.1 SELF COMPASSION

About six months after finishing my training and entering into practice, I had a run of surgical complications. Most of them were minor: seromas, incision infections, and the like. However, they were really doing a number on my self-confidence. My previous confidence in my surgical skills was rapidly declining, and I began to wonder if I was a bad surgeon.

I finally mustered the courage to approach one of my mentors. She gave me some very practical advice on closing techniques to prevent seromas, but the pep talk she gave me was far more impactful. She started by walking me through my case numbers. Since entering practice, I was doing a lot more surgeries than I did during my training. She then emphasized that anyone who does surgery is going to have complications. No one likes complications, but they are just a fact of life as a surgeon. She then told me that having complications didn't make me a bad doctor. What was more important was how I chose to deal with them, and by acknowledging that I was having complications and seeking mentorship, I had shown that I was a good doctor who cared about my results. Her advice really helped me. I was finally able to let go of some of the shame and panic I was feeling and started to focus on how I could improve my surgical skills. I'm grateful to her to this day. Even a decade later, I think about that conversation when I have a complication. It helps me remind myself that complications happen, and how we grow from them matters more.

BOUNDARIES

"Boundaries are like the ropes at the museum that keep every eager visitor at a safe distance to preserve the masterpiece and allow the visitors to enjoy the art" (Mammoliti 2022).

Boundaries are not barriers, but safeguards that preserve well-being and allow for authentic connection. The APA defines a boundary as a "psychological demarcation that protects the integrity of an individual or group" (APA 2018). In veterinary medicine, where emotional labor and client demands often overlap, boundaries are essential for sustainable and ethical practice.

Poor boundary management has been described as an "unrecognized risk for burnout," and it remains an understudied area in healthcare wellness (Thomas 2019, pg. 998). The challenge lies in balancing compassion with professional distance. Clinical empathy is vital, but unmodulated, it can lead to overinvolvement. Blurred personal-professional roles like excessive self-disclosure, being asked for medical advice by friends outside of the clinic, or responding to client contact outside of work hours are common boundary-crossing behaviors in healthcare (Lampe et al. 2023). These behaviors may feel caring, but can foster emotional fatigue and erode accountability.

Healthy limits require awareness and practice. Nedra Tawwab (2021), licensed therapist and author of *Set Boundaries, Find Peace*, recommends identifying one's boundaries, stating needs clearly, and accepting the discomfort that often accompanies self-advocacy. Ultimately, boundaries support not only clinician well-being but also client care, fostering clarity, consistency, and genuine compassion (Chernata 2024). Nedra Tawwab's books and podcasts are excellent resources for those seeking to work on their boundaries.

MINDFULNESS

Mindfulness is the practice of paying attention with calm, nonjudgmental awareness – being present to both internal states and external surroundings. Rooted in Buddhist and Hindu traditions, it was adapted into modern clinical practice by Jon Kabat-Zinn through Mindfulness-Based Stress Reduction (MBSR) in the late 1970s (Kabat-Zinn 2013; Selva 2017). Crucially, mindfulness involves observing thoughts and feelings without judgment, fostering awareness that leads to acceptance rather than self-criticism (Bishop et al. 2004).

Common introductory techniques include the body scan, which directs attention sequentially through the body, and breathing practices that focus on pacing or rhythm. Box breathing is one such technique, involving a repeated cycle of inhaling for four seconds, holding for four seconds, exhaling for four seconds, and holding again for four seconds. Both meditation and breathwork reduce negative affect and anxiety while increasing positive affect, and recent evidence suggests breathwork may be especially effective (Balban et al. 2023). These findings are reinforced by a meta-analysis of 419 studies and over 53,000 participants, which found mindfulness consistently improved mental well-being, with even greater benefits in individuals with mental illness (van Agteren 2021).

Mindfulness also need not be our only coping skill; instead, it should be viewed as one tool in a toolbox. The practice of nonjudgmental self-awareness can help assess which other techniques might be beneficial, and mindfulness has shown benefit when combined with other interventions. For instance, integrating mindfulness with self-compassion techniques has proven particularly effective in addressing self-criticism and perfectionism, which are common challenges in veterinary medicine (Wakelin 2021).

There are a plethora of resources for those wishing to learn more about mindfulness. Examples include Dan Harris' book *10% Happier*, as well as an app and podcast of the same name. Other popular mindfulness apps include Headspace, Calm, Insight Timer, and Mindfulness Coach. Jon Kabat-Zinn, who first adapted the practice of mindfulness to modern clinical practice, also has several books on the subject, including *Wherever You Go, There You Are* and *Mindfulness for Beginners*. If you are just getting started, it's important to remind yourself that it's called "mindfulness practice" for a reason. Mindfulness is a skill that you aren't likely to be very good at the first couple of times you try it, and if you don't connect with one practice, there are many different ways to practice mindfulness. One good starting point, recommended by Dr. Marsha Linehan, the developer of Dialectical Behavior Therapy (Linehan 1993), is to try using mindfulness while doing a routine chore, like the dishes. Notice and describe, nonjudgmentally, the temperature of the water, the scent of the soap, the sound of the pots and pans clanking, and the rainbow colors in the bubbles. Just be in the moment, not thinking of all the other things you could or should be doing. In Story 10.2, a veterinarian describes how, after some failed attempts, they found a way to practice mindfulness daily. Build a simple mindfulness practice into your daily routine, so it becomes familiar and more natural for you, and when you encounter the stresses of daily life, your body and mind are prepared to put the skill to use.

GRATITUDE, HOPE, AND OPTIMISM

Gratitude, hope, and optimism are closely linked yet distinct traits within positive psychology. Gratitude grounds us in appreciation of the present, optimism reflects general expectations of positive outcomes, and hope adds agency and pathways to pursue goals despite obstacles (Emmons and McCullough 2003; Dursun 2021). Together, they foster resilience, support well-being, and help individuals navigate adversity. Research shows their strong impact; in one study of 510 university students, gratitude, hope, optimism, and life satisfaction explained over half the variance in psychological well-being, with gratitude alone accounting for more than a third (Kardaş et al. 2019).

Interventions show these dispositions can be strengthened: goal-setting and agency-building enhance hope, and training hope has been shown to reduce burnout and secondary traumatic stress in healthcare workers (Pharris 2025). Similarly, gratitude exercises, such as the Three Good Things exercise, have been shown in double-blind randomized controlled trials to reduce perceived stress and depressive symptoms in health care workers (Cheng et al. 2015).

STORY 10.2 MOVING MINDFULNESS

When I first started working on my mental health, I did what many people do and downloaded a mindfulness app. I dutifully opened the first exercise, where a very calm voice guided me through a body scan, naming each body part in turn and asking me to rest my attention there.

It was torture. I have attention-deficit hyperactivity disorder (ADHD), and sitting still has never come naturally to me, particularly when paired with silent inward reflection. I did not expect instant success, so I kept trying the exercises for a few weeks, but eventually I concluded that this simply was not for me.

I later described this abject failure to my therapist. Her first response was: "You don't have to do mindfulness. There are lots of other things we can work on." She even joked that she would happily write me a note excusing me from mindfulness if it helped me let myself off the hook. Then she added that there is more than one way to learn this skill, if seated meditation wasn't doing it for me.

As she described different approaches, the idea of moving meditation came up. I realized that, unintentionally, I was already practicing mindfulness skills. At the time, I was training for a race, which meant paying close attention to my body as I pushed myself to go faster and further than I had before. During my morning runs, I spent 30 minutes focusing on posture, leg movement, breathing patterns, and checking in with my body for any signs of discomfort. Was I tired? Do these shoes hurt? I would spend a minute or two at a time noting the exact way my foot hit the ground.

That practice turned out to be mindfulness, just delivered in a format my brain could tolerate. From there, I extended the skill into other areas of my life.

You may recall in the first chapter of this book (Story 1.2), a veterinarian implemented the Three Good Things exercise and how it helped her improve her coping skills when her practice had a water leak. Previously a pessimistic person, the implementation of this gratitude exercise gave her the skills to see the tiny bright spots in an otherwise terrible situation. Appreciating small things, like being grateful to her custodian for contacting her about the leak and for having the things she needed to address it already on hand, helped her emotionally regulate and work on problem-solving. This shift in perspective is also the foundation of another helpful coping strategy known as positive reframing.

COGNITIVE REAPPRAISAL AND POSITIVE REFRAMING

Cognitive reappraisal is a core emotion-regulation strategy first described within cognitive theory in the 1960s, later formalized in cognitive behavioral therapy (Beck 1964, 1976). Reappraisal involves deliberately reconsidering how one interprets a situation to moderate the emotions related to the event. Positive reframing is a form of cognitive reappraisal focused specifically on more balanced or optimistic appraisals, including identifying meaning, learning, or small successes under challenging circumstances (Folkman and Moskowitz 2000).

In veterinary medicine, studies show that cognitive reappraisal is a common and valuable coping strategy, and survey data links its use with lower emotional exhaustion and better well-being (Bostock et al., 2018). A qualitative study of veterinarians found that structured reflection helped clinicians re-evaluate emotionally charged events – such as medical errors or client conflict – and shift from guilt and anxiety toward more balanced interpretations and greater confidence (Kinnison and May 2017). In Story 10.3, a veterinarian shares a technique she learned that helps her step out of judgment and self-criticism. Instead of treating the inner voice of "I'm terrible at this" as fact, she paused, examined the evidence, and reframed the situation realistically: a single complication did not mean she was a bad surgeon – just a good surgeon who had a bad day.

STORY 10.3 PUTTING THINGS IN CONTEXT

I used to be a world champion at beating myself up. If anything went wrong with a case, even something minor, it would send me straight into a tailspin of self-doubt and self-criticism.

Sure enough, I had a major complication during a surgery, and I was upset and very focused on every little thing I should have done better. I was telling my therapist about this and how scared I was to ever do this surgery again, or frankly, any surgery at all. She asked me, "How many of those surgeries have you done?" For that particular surgery, the answer was a lot. Easily a hundred in the last few years. "And this is the only one you can remember going wrong?" I confirmed that. "So, if we do the math, you have greater than a 99% success rate."

That was so helpful to me. It helped me get out of the doom spiral where I was beating myself up. The math was clear. I had a 99% success rate, and it was factually untrue that I was bad at my job, despite what that little voice in my head wanted to tell me. I wasn't a bad surgeon; I was a good surgeon who had a bad day. I asked her some time later, "What happens if I haven't done hundreds?" "Well, you can't really expect yourself to be perfect at something you are learning now, can you?"

And I still use that technique to this day. When I start beating myself up, I take a breath and do the math. Looking at the facts lets me let go of all of those unhelpful, perfectionist, and negative thoughts. It allows me to calm down and start doing more helpful things, like analyzing what I could have done better and learning from the experience.

That simple act of stepping back reduced emotional intensity, allowed learning, and prevented a spiral of perfectionistic self-blame.

Clinical narratives similarly describe veterinarians reframing complex cases by recognizing what was within their control, identifying positive elements of care, and extracting learning points, an approach linked with improved psychological functioning (White 2018). Although the evidence base is still developing, these findings mirror broader healthcare research showing that reappraisal predicts lower stress and stronger resilience in demanding clinical settings (Troy et al. 2010).

Cognitive reappraisal is a learnable skill. Mindfulness can help clinicians notice automatic thoughts as they arise, evaluate whether those thoughts are accurate or helpful, and generate alternative interpretations (Beck 2011). Story 10.3 offers a practical example of a veterinarian using this approach to shift away from self-criticism and regain perspective. Several resources include books such as *Feeling Good* by David D. Burns and *Mind Over Mood* by Dennis Greenberger and Christine A. Padesky, which offer structured exercises for practicing cognitive reappraisal.

PHYSICAL SELF-CARE

It feels patronizing to remind medical professionals of the importance of sleep, exercise, and hydration – we are trained at a cellular level in these fundamentals. Yet this knowledge does not always translate into healthy behaviors. Despite their expertise, 57% of healthcare workers report sleep deprivation, and 41% of doctors and nurses finish shifts dehydrated to the point of oliguria (El-Sharkawy et al. 2016; Hattatoğlu et al. 2020). If those who routinely calculate fluid requirements and measure urine outputs for their patients cannot personally maintain adequate hydration to preserve their own renal functions, it is clear that knowledge alone is insufficient.

The key lies in planning and habit-building. Knowing you should drink water is different from bringing a bottle to work and keeping it within reach. This is an area where mentorship can play an excellent role. With extended clinic hours, busy schedules, and a host of other competing demands, exactly how we can achieve things like exercise and healthy eating can seem an insurmountable task. However, solutions can often be found in discussions with more experienced professionals.

Exercise is another form of physical self-care. Exercise has been shown to have not only an impact on physical health but also on mental health and well-being. In one study, healthy adults not only showed improvements in positive affect over controls after exercise but also exhibited different neural responses to both positive and stressful stimuli on functional magnetic resonance imaging (fMRI). The results suggested that after exercise, the brain is more open to positive emotions and is better at both filtering and processing negative emotions (Ligeza et al. 2023). One study showed that people who exercise regularly experience on average 34.5% fewer days of poor mental health per month compared with those who do not exercise (Chekroud et al. 2018). In Story 10.4, a veterinarian discusses how she fits in exercise and the importance that it has had on her well-being in addition to her physical health.

As alluded to by the veterinarian in Story 10.4, exercise is an effective intervention for both depression and anxiety, with outcomes comparable to established treatments such as psychotherapy or medication. A recent network meta-analysis (Noetel et al. 2024) found that various forms of exercise are moderately effective treatments for depression, with greater benefits at higher intensities. Exercise also improved the outcomes of traditional selective serotonin reuptake inhibitor (SSRI) therapy when the two were combined. Similarly, a meta-analysis of randomized controlled trials demonstrated that exercise produces small-to-moderate reductions in anxiety symptoms, with aerobic and moderate-to-vigorous intensity programs yielding the strongest effects (Ramos-Sanchez et al. 2021).

Veterinary medicine is a very physical profession, and our rates of injury are notably high. This makes physical self-care particularly important in our profession. While no amount of exercise can prevent a cat bite or a horse kick, it can help prevent things like back strains (Huang et al. 2020). Physical self-care also needs to include rest and recovery when we are sick or injured in order to have a full recovery. Investing time in rest rather than pushing through can help you recover more fully and quickly to show up as the clinician you want to be. Unfortunately, taking time off can sometimes be difficult. In a survey of Australian veterinarians, 24.6% (n = 18) felt they would be unlikely to be able to take sick leave at short notice, and many vet professionals, especially in support staff roles, cannot afford to take time off (Hilton et al. 2023). This emphasizes the importance of organizational-level support for well-being.

STORY 10.4 EXERCISE AND WELLBEING

When I was in vet school, I injured my back picking up a dog. The only time I could fit in physical therapy was very early in the morning, before rotations started. I certainly didn't relish getting up even earlier, but these appointments led to a discovery that has had a long-term impact on my well-being. I noticed that on the days I got up early and did my exercises, I felt better – not just physically, but also mentally. My anxiety was more manageable. I was more focused and just felt better overall. I was happier, which was a bit of a surprise. I expected to be physically stronger and to be in less pain, but I didn't expect the mental health aspects.

I knew that working out was good for me, and I had been relatively consistent with exercise during my undergraduate training. However, with the extra stress and time commitment of vet school, I had fallen out of the habit. Too often, clinic duties left me too exhausted at the end of the day to even fathom going to the gym. Without that push from physical therapy, I also would have thought that the hours of sleep I miss would, on balance, negate the effects of working out for me, but that just didn't turn out to be the case. Don't get me wrong, I still groan when the alarm goes off at 5:00 am. But the knowledge that staying strong will protect me from further injury and the mental health benefits of exercise have made me get out of bed early for 20 years.

Not all aspects of physical well-being are entirely under our control, such as severe and chronic illnesses. Illness has a well-recognized impact on well-being (Wiseman et al. 2016; Lim 2020). However, research has shown that implementing other self-care strategies can help balance out the negative well-being effects. In a review, numerous practices such as gratitude exercises and mindfulness reduced stress and fostered resilience across patients with chronic illness (Ghosh and Deb 2017). Additionally, the presence of an illness does not preclude the use of other physical self-care. For example, in women with chronic illness, physical activity was linked to lower depression scores (Mcintyre et al., 2019). These findings further illustrate the importance of a diversity of self-care strategies both within and between the domains of self-care.

OCCUPATIONAL SELF-CARE

Chapters 6 and 7 have an extensive review of various aspects of our occupation that can either be supportive or detrimental to our well-being. However, one area that we have not yet explored in depth is the importance of growth and development. This element of our well-being, closely tied to both occupational and intellectual self-care, was identified as one of the two key factors in professional happiness in a review of veterinary well-being literature and therefore deserves attention (Cake et al., 2015). Central to professional development is a growth mindset or the belief that our abilities are "malleable and improvable" (Ng 2018).

People with a growth mindset are more likely to use active coping strategies and report lower levels of psychological distress (Burnette et al. 2020). Without this foundational belief, the motivation to pursue positive change can falter. In Story 10.1, the young veterinarian initially adopts a fixed mindset. She was focusing on the complications and concluding that she was a bad surgeon rather than engaging in proactive problem-focused coping. However, after speaking with her mentor and receiving some advice around self-compassion, she was able to reframe her challenges. Instead of believing that her complications made her a bad surgeon, she was able to see that how she dealt with her challenges was what mattered most. This led her to a growth mindset, which allowed her to improve her skills. This example shows us that active coping strategies, such as positive reframing, can help shift us into more effective problem-oriented coping strategies and protect our well-being.

SELF-EFFICACY

Closely linked to a growth mindset is self-efficacy or the belief in one's ability to manage challenges and access necessary resources. It is not only the belief that growth is possible but also the belief that one can personally achieve that growth. In a study of 800 veterinarians, those with high self-efficacy showed greater resilience and lower stress (McArthur et al. 2021). Similarly, research with Iranian nurses found that self-efficacy buffered the effects of occupational stress on mental health (Rafiei et al. 2024). In high-pressure environments, confidence in one's ability to act is often the first step in reducing the psychological burden of stress.

Self-efficacy is not an all-or-nothing quality; it is domain-specific. A clinician may feel highly competent managing a difficult client, but less comfortable in surgery or research. Identifying these domains offers both a roadmap for playing to strengths and a clear starting point for growth. Structured goals also provide direction and increase confidence, making stressful situations more manageable (Rafiei et al. 2024).

Importantly, evidence in veterinary medicine shows that self-efficacy can be developed. A one-year development program for recent veterinary graduates increased self-efficacy, proactive behavior, and reflective practice (Mastenbroek et al. 2015). Shorter interventions are helpful as well. In veterinary students, brief health promotion micro-breaks improved self-efficacy in caring for their physical and emotional well-being during training (Grünwald et al. 2023). Improvements are not limited to those new to a field: academic clinicians with formal research training reported significantly higher research self-efficacy than those without it (Moore and O'Kell 2024). Together, these findings suggest that self-efficacy is not fixed; it grows with support, skill development, and opportunities for mastery.

GOAL-SETTING

Belief must eventually lead to action. One of the most effective ways to bridge that gap is through goal-setting. Teaching people how to set and plan for goals has been shown to causally improve well-being (MacLeod et al. 2008). Goal-setting and growth mindsets mutually reinforce one another as growth mindsets promote intrinsic motivation by helping people perceive value and enjoyment in self-improvement in and of itself, rather than just the rewards of that improvement (Ng 2018). Growth mindsets also help individuals view setbacks and incremental progress as part of the learning process, which increases motivation and resilience. So a growth mindset allows us to both enjoy the learning process and stick with our goals. In turn, as we achieve and celebrate our progress, it enhances well-being by improving intrinsic motivation and strengthening the belief that growth is possible (Ng 2018).

So, with the belief that we can improve in mind, we start by setting a goal. Structured goal-setting techniques help break large challenges into achievable steps, making progress visible and sustainable. One widely used and evidence-supported method is the SMART goal framework, which encourages goals to be specific, measurable, achievable, relevant, and time-bound (Aghera et al. 2017). An example of using the SMART goal framework is provided in Table 10.1.

Table 10.1 Applying SMART goals: a practical example

Consider a large, aspirational goal: *Become proficient in orthopedic surgery*. While admirable, this goal is too vague to act on. Let's break it down using the SMART framework, focusing on cranial cruciate ligament repair via TPLO surgery:

- Specific: I want to become proficient at performing TPLO surgeries. This means I feel comfortable planning and performing the procedure unsupervised and have a good handle on how to handle common complications.
- Measurable: I will complete 12 TPLO surgeries under mentor supervision, followed by five independently.
- Achievable: My coworker is proficient in TPLO surgeries, and is willing to mentor me.
- Relevant: I enjoy surgery and want to build skills that align with my career goals.
- Time-bound: I will complete this goal within the next 12 months.

This structured approach transforms an intimidating aspiration into an actionable plan—promoting both confidence and progress.

Research participants who used SMART goal-setting strategies reported improved goal attainment, higher psychological need satisfaction, and increased positive affect in comparison to controls who did not receive instruction on goal-setting (Bahrami et al. 2022).

Framing goals around meaningful work, such as improving patient care, mentoring colleagues, or supporting the team, can enhance their positive impact on well-being by reinforcing professional identity and purpose (Wallace 2019).

SPIRITUAL SELF-CARE

While religion and spirituality share several principles, they are distinct entities. Religion refers to the formal and outward expression of faith, often through the beliefs and practices of a specific religious tradition. Spirituality, by contrast, is a more personal search for meaning, transcendence, and interconnectedness, which may occur within or outside organized religion (Lim 2015; Willani 2019).

In a large meta-analysis, both religion and spirituality showed positive impacts on well-being, particularly life satisfaction, with spirituality having the greater impact (r = 0.30 vs 0.16; Yaden et al. 2022). In several studies, religious attendance is also positively correlated with well-being measures, with those attending more often experiencing greater benefits. This is particularly true in cultures and religions that are more observant and consider religion an important part of life (Lim 2015; Yaden et al. 2022). Religion and spirituality are thought to support well-being through a variety of mechanisms, including social support; positive identity, additional coping mechanisms; increased sense of control, increased positive emotions, including hope and optimism, and a sense of meaning and purpose (Koenig 2012; Aggarwal et al. 2023). Of the various aspects of spirituality, this sense of meaning and purpose has the strongest impact on well-being across populations, and this holds in veterinary medicine as well (Cake 2015; Villani et al. 2019).

Throughout this textbook, we have discussed numerous challenges professionals face. A majority of veterinary professionals face difficult questions and situations on a daily basis (Kipperman et al. 2017). Veterinarians average ~7.5 euthanasias per month (Dickinson et al. 2011), and most report grief responses when an animal dies (86.7%; Pohl et al. 2022), suggesting grief is a routine part of clinical life. Spirituality, particularly the dimensions of meaning and purpose, can buffer the well-being risks inherent in work that routinely exposes clinicians to grief, moral distress, and potentially traumatizing events (Batchelor and McKeegan 2012; Moses et al. 2018; Kogan and Rishniw 2023; Gaur 2025). This protective effect is recognized across healthcare settings, with higher spiritual well-being and a clearer sense of meaning consistently associated with lower compassion fatigue, burnout, and moral injury in human health care (Hooker et al. 2020; D'Alessandro-Lowe 2023). It's no wonder that Cake et al. (2015) found that a sense of meaning and purpose was essential to happiness in our field.

THE CORE OF MEANINGFUL WORK

According to Martela and Pessi (2018), meaningful work is grounded in significance, the perception that one's efforts matter. This significance can be achieved through two primary pathways: self-realization, which involves personal growth and alignment with one's values, and purpose, which connects the work to broader, often moral or societal, and goals. One need not look far for purpose in this field. There are numerous avenues that range from healing the sick and helping those in need to supporting public health. Unsurprisingly, the importance of meaning has been echoed by other researchers in the field of veterinary well-being. In a survey of 376 veterinary workers, it was once again confirmed that team belonging (discussed in Chapter 7), self-actualization, and meaningful work were positively correlated with well-being (Wallace 2019). Moreover, specific aspects of their work, such as helping animals, supporting clients, and having a strong connection to their professional identity, contributed significantly to the perceived meaning of the work. However, as with other dimensions of self-care, the buffering role of meaningful work is not, on its own, sufficient to negate all stressors. Importantly, Wallace (2019) found that certain stressors, such as financial concerns and workload, were not effectively buffered by meaningful work. This once again highlights the importance of a multifaceted approach to well-being and self-care.

RETHINKING WORK TO ENHANCE MEANING

While purpose and meaning are readily available in veterinary medicine, the day-to-day grind can disconnect us from accessing them. Wallace (2019) suggests three places professionals can re-examine their work to connect to meaning: shared narratives, job roles, and relationships.

The way we think and talk about tasks shapes our perception of them. By promoting a shared narrative where every role – from reception to surgery – is essential to meaningful goals like animal health, we help create an environment of meaning and purpose. There are plenty of dirty, seemingly menial tasks in veterinary medicine. In and of themselves, these tasks are hardly glamorous. Take cleaning cages. Cleaning up bodily fluids is unlikely to give one a deep sense of purpose, and it would be easy to belittle the individual in the clinic charged with doing it. However, this task is no less important to the health of your patients than the most intricate of surgical procedures. Without clean cages, the patients would be uncomfortable and dirty. The environment of the clinic would be unbearable for the staff. Infections would be out of control. So we can reframe that task (and cleaning in general) as patient care and infection control. This helps connect the routine, unpleasant task to the greater purpose and meaning of the job: helping animals and promoting health.

Of course, crafty wordsmithing alone is not enough. As much as possible, it's important that we ensure every role has an opportunity to engage with tasks central to the core mission. For instance, a manager's duties are largely administrative tasks that keep them shuttered in the office for the majority of the day. However, they can attend patient rounds every morning, not only to connect with the team, but also to remind themselves that all of those administrative tasks help support these patients.

Finally, it's important to work on our relationships, both within our team and with the profession as a whole. This could take the form of taking a moment to recognize and thank a coworker for their contribution. It could also mean volunteering with various professional organizations or nonprofits to foster a sense of belonging and greater purpose.

INTELLECTUAL SELF-CARE

Even within our patient populations, we recognize the importance of intellectual stimulation for well-being to the point that cognitive enrichment is a requirement for accreditation by organizations like the Association of Zoos and Aquariums (Association of Zoos and Aquariums 2025). It is no surprise that cognitive enrichment is equally important to humans. The opportunity to learn and enhance our own skills is an important, if not key, factor in veterinary well-being. It significantly protects against burnout and encourages work engagement in veterinary technicians (Kimber and Gardner 2016; Kogan et al. 2020). In a sample of 860 Dutch veterinarians, professional development predicted work engagement (Mastenbroek et al. 2014). In fact, in a comprehensive review of veterinary well-being, Cake et al. (2015) found that the two largest predictors of positive well-being in the veterinary profession were meaningful purpose and self-development. Much of the well-being literature discusses professional development as a means to deliver information on well-being skills, yet the process of learning itself appears intrinsically protective.

It's fitting that we close our textbook with intellectual self-care. We hope that the material presented in this text has not only offered an opportunity for stimulation and reflection, but also equipped you with knowledge and tools to enhance your own well-being and to support the well-being of your peers.

REFERENCES

Adin, D.B., Royal, K.D. and Adin, C.A. (2020) 'Cross-sectional assessment of the emotional intelligence of fourth-year veterinary students and veterinary house officers in a teaching hospital', *Journal of Veterinary Medical Education*, 47(2), pp. 193–201. DOI: https://doi.org/10.3138/jvme.0518-065r.

Aggarwal, S., Wright, J., Morgan, A. et al. (2023). Religiosity and spirituality in the prevention and management of depression and anxiety in young people: a systematic review and meta-analysis. *BMC Psychiatry* 23 (1): 729.

Aghera, A., Emery, M., Bounds, R. et al. (2017). A randomized trial of SMART goal enhanced debriefing after simulation to promote educational actions. *Western Journal of Emergency Medicine* 19 (1): 112.

American Psychological Association (2018) 'Boundary'. APA Dictionary of Psychology. Available at: https://dictionary.apa.org/boundary (Accessed: 28 March 2026).

Association of Zoos and Aquariums (2025). *Accreditation Standards & Related Policies: 2025 Edition* (ed. Association of Zoos and Aquariums) section 1.5.0, 18–19. Silver Spring, MD.

Asuero, A.M., Queraltó, J.M., Pujol-Ribera, E. et al. (2014). Effectiveness of a mindfulness education program in primary health care professionals: a pragmatic controlled trial. *Journal of Continuing Education in the Health Professions* 34 (1): 4–12.

Bahrami, Z., Heidari, A., and Cranney, J. (2022). Applying SMART Goal Intervention Leads to Greater Goal Attainment, Need Satisfaction and Positive Affect. *International Journal of Mental Health Promotion* 24 (6): 869–882.

Balban, M.Y., Neri, E., Kogon, M.M. et al. (2023). Brief structured respiration practices enhance mood and reduce physiological arousal. *Cell Reports Medicine* 4 (1): 1–10.

Batchelor, C.E.M. and McKeegan, D.E.F. (2012). Survey of the frequency and perceived stressfulness of ethical dilemmas encountered in UK veterinary practice. *Veterinary Record* 170 (1): 19–19.

Beck, A.T. (1964). Thinking and depression: II. Theory and therapy. *Archives of general psychiatry* 10 (6): 561–571.

Beck, A.T., 1976. Cognitive therapy and the emotional disorders. 1976. American book, New-York. p213–229

Beck, J.S. (2011) *Cognitive Behavior Therapy: Basics and Beyond*. 2nd edn. New York: Guilford Press.

Bishop, S.R., Lau, M., Shapiro, S. et al. (2004). Mindfulness: A proposed operational definition. *Clinical psychology: Science and practice* 11 (3): 230–241.

Bostock, R., Kinnison, T., and May, S.A. (2018). Mindset and its relationship to anxiety in clinical veterinary students. *Veterinary Record* 183 (20): 623–623.

Bradberry, T. and Greaves, J. (2009). *Emotional Intelligence 2.0*. San Diego: TalentSmart.

Burnette, J.L., Pollack, J.M., Forsyth, R.B. et al. (2020). A growth mindset intervention: Enhancing students' entrepreneurial self-efficacy and career development. *Entrepreneurship Theory and Practice* 44 (5): 878–908.

Cake, M.A., Bell, M.A., Bickley, N., and Bartram, D.J. (2015). The life of meaning: a model of the positive contributions to well-being from veterinary work. *Journal of veterinary medical education* 42 (3): 184–193.

Chekroud, S.R., Gueorguieva, R., Zheutlin, A.B. et al. (2018). Association between physical exercise and mental health in 1·2 million individuals in the USA between 2011 and 2015: a cross-sectional study. *Lancet Psychiatry* 5 (9): 739–746.

Cheng, S.T., Tsui, P.K., and Lam, J.H. (2015). Improving mental health in health care practitioners: randomized controlled trial of a gratitude intervention. *Journal of Consulting and Clinical Psychology* 83 (1): 177.

Chernata, T. (2024). Personal boundaries: definition, role, and impact on mental health. *Personality and environmental issues* 3 (1): 24–30.

Ciarrochi, J., Hayes, S.C., Oades, L.G., and Hofmann, S.G. (2022). Toward a unified framework for positive psychology interventions: evidence-based processes of change in coaching, prevention, and training. *Frontiers in Psychology* 12: 809362.

D'Alessandro-Lowe, A.M., Karram, M., Ritchie, K. et al. (2023). Coping, supports and moral injury: Spiritual well-being and organizational support are associated with reduced moral injury in Canadian healthcare providers during the COVID-19 pandemic. *International journal of environmental research and public health* 20 (19): 6812.

Deslippe, A.L., Soanes, A., Bouchaud, C.C. et al. (2023). Barriers and facilitators to diet, physical activity and lifestyle behavior intervention adherence: a qualitative systematic review of the literature. *International Journal of Behavioral Nutrition and Physical Activity* 20 (1): 14.

Dickinson, G.E., Roof, P.D., and Roof, K.W. (2011). A survey of veterinarians in the US: Euthanasia and other end-of-life issues. *Anthrozoös* 24 (2): 167–174.

Dorociak, K.E., 2015. Development of the personal and professional self-care scale. Master's thesis. Loyola University Chicago.

Dursun, P. (2021). Optimism, hope and subjective well-being: a literature overview. *Çatalhöyük Uluslararası Turizm ve Sosyal Araştırmalar Dergisi* 6: 61–74.

El-Sharkawy, A.M., Bragg, D., Watson, P. et al. (2016). Hydration amongst nurses and doctors on-call (the HANDS on prospective cohort study). *Clinical Nutrition* 35 (4): 935–942.

Emmons, R.A. and McCullough, M.E. (2003). Counting blessings versus burdens: an experimental investigation of gratitude and subjective well-being in daily life. *Journal of Personality and Social Psychology* 84 (2): 377.

Folkman, S. and Moskowitz, J.T. (2000). Positive affect and the other side of coping. *American psychologist* 55 (6): 647.

Gardner, B., Lally, P., and Wardle, J. (2012). Making health habitual: the psychology of 'habit-formation' and general practice. *The British Journal of General Practice* 62 (605): 664.

Gaur, K., 2025. Meaning-making in grief work and where we stand today. *Illness, Crisis & Loss*, 34(2), 209–238 p.https://doi.org/10.1177/10541373251318126.

Ghosh, A. and Deb, A. (2017). Positive psychology interventions for chronic physical illnesses: A systematic review. *Psychological Studies* 62 (3): 213–232.

Grimani, A., Aboagye, E., and Kwak, L. (2019). The effectiveness of workplace nutrition and physical activity interventions in improving productivity, work performance and workability: a systematic review. *BMC Public Health* 19 (1): 1676.

Grünwald, J.A. and Licka, T.F. (2023). Health promotion for students of veterinary medicine: a preliminary study on active microbreaks and ergonomics education. *Animals* 13 (10): 1641.

Hattatoğlu, D.G., Aydin, Ş., Aydin, C., and Yildiz, B.P. (2020). The effect of sleep hygiene and sleep deterioration on quality of life in shiftworking healthcare professionals. *Archives of Neuropsychiatry* 58 (1): 11.

Hernández-Esteve, I., Zumbado, M., and Henríquez-Hernández, L.A. (2024). Burnout and mental health among veterinarians: the role of self-compassion and associated risk factors. *Veterinary Record* 196 (5): e4960.

Hilton, K.R., Burke, K.J., and Signal, T. (2023). Mental health in the veterinary profession: an individual or organisational focus? *Australian Veterinary Journal* 101 (1-2): 41–48.

Hodzic, S., Scharfen, J., Ripoll, P. et al. (2018). How efficient are emotional intelligence trainings: a meta-analysis. *Emotion Review* 10 (2): 138–148.

Holden, C.L. (2020). Characteristics of veterinary students: perfectionism, personality factors, and resilience. *Journal of Veterinary Medical Education* 47 (4): 488–496.

Hooker, S., Post, R., and Sherman, M. (2020). Awareness of meaning in life is protective against burnout among family physicians: a CERA study. *Family medicine* 52 (1): 11–16.

Huang, R., Ning, J., Chuter, V.H. et al. (2020). Exercise alone and exercise combined with education both prevent episodes of low back pain and related absenteeism: systematic review and network meta-analysis of randomised controlled trials (RCTs) aimed at preventing back pain. *British Journal of Sports Medicine* 54 (13): 766–770.

James, W. (1892). The conscious self. In: *The Principles of Psychology*, vol. 1), Chapter 10. Cambridge, MA: Harvard University Press.

Kabat-Zinn, J. (2013). *Full Catastrophe Living, Revised Edition: How to Cope with Stress, Pain and Illness Using Mindfulness Meditation*. New York: Hachette UK.

Karaffa, K.M., Hancock, T.S., and Sanford-Martens, T.C. (2024). Perfectionistic cognitions, self-compassion, and psychological distress among veterinary students. *Journal of College Student Mental Health* 39: 1–24.

Kardas, F., Cam, Z., Eskısu, M., and Gelıbolu, S. (2019). Gratitude, hope, optimism and life satisfaction as predictors of psychological well-being. *Eurasian Journal of Educational Research* 19 (82): 81–100.

Keyes, J., Yankouskaya, A. and Panourgia, C. (2022) 'Self-compassion, coping strategies and gender differences in psychology, counselling and psychotherapy practitioners during COVID-19: Lessons learnt', Counselling and Psychotherapy Research. doi: https://doi.org/10.1002/capr.12574.

Kimber, S. and Gardner, D.H. (2016). Relationships between workplace well-being, job demands and resources in a sample of veterinary nurses in New Zealand. *New Zealand veterinary journal* 64 (4): 224–229.

Kinnison, T. and May, S. (2017). Continuing professional development: researching non-technical competencies can support cognitive reappraisal and reduced stress in clinicians. *Veterinary Record* 181 (10): 266–266.

Kipperman, B.S., Kass, P.H., and Rishniw, M. (2017). Factors that influence small animal veterinarians' opinions and actions regarding cost of care and effects of economic limitations on patient care and outcome and professional career satisfaction and burnout. *Journal of the American Veterinary Medical Association* 250 (7): 785–794.

Koenig, H.G. (2012). Religion, spirituality, and health: the research and clinical implications. *International Scholarly Research Notices* 2012 (1): 278730.

Kogan, L.R. and Rishniw, M. (2023). Veterinarians and moral distress. *Journal of the American Veterinary Medical Association* 261 (5): 1–7.

Kogan, L.R., Rishniw, M., Hellyer, P.W., and Schoenfeld-Tacher, R.M. (2018). Veterinarians' experiences with near misses and adverse events. *Journal of the American Veterinary Medical Association* 252 (5): 586–595.

Kogan, L.R., Wallace, J.E., Schoenfeld-Tacher, R. et al. (2020). Veterinary technicians and occupational burnout. *Frontiers in Veterinary Science* 7: 328.

Lampe, L., Hitching, R., Hammond, T.E. et al. (2023). Being a 'good' doctor: understanding and managing professional boundaries is challenging and can lead to stress and burnout. *Australasian Psychiatry* 31 (6): 764–767.

Lazarus, R.S. (1984). *Stress, appraisal, and coping*, vol. 445. New York, NY: Springer.

Leipold, B., Klier, K., Dapperger, E., and Schmidt, A. (2024). Physical activity and nutrition in relation to resilience: a cross-sectional study. *Scientific Reports* 14 (1): 2272.

Ligeza, T.S., Maciejczyk, M., Wyczesany, M., and Junghofer, M. (2023). The effects of a single aerobic exercise session on mood and neural emotional reactivity in depressed and healthy young adults: A late positive potential study. *Psychophysiology* 60 (1): e14137.

Lim, C. (2015). Religion and subjective well-being across religious traditions: evidence from 1.3 million Americans. *Journal for the Scientific Study of Religion* 54 (4): 684–701.

Lim, S.S. (2020). The effects of chronic illness on aspirations and subjective wellbeing. *Journal of Happiness Studies* 21 (5): 1771–1793.

Linehan, M. (1993). *Cognitive-Behavioral Treatment of Borderline Personality Disorder*. New York: Guilford press.

López-López, V., Lagos San Martín, N., Cabello Gonzalez, R., et al. (2025) 'Transversal education in higher education: a study on emotional competencies and emotional intelligence in Veterinary Medicine and Nursing', *Salud, Ciencia y Tecnología*, 5, p. 1150. DOI: https://doi.org/10.56294/saludcyt20251150.

Lyubomirsky, S., Sheldon, K.M., and Schkade, D. (2005). Pursuing happiness: The architecture of sustainable change. *Review of general psychology* 9 (2): 111–131.

MacLeod, A.K., Coates, E., and Hetherton, J. (2008). Increasing well-being through teaching goal-setting and planning skills: Results of a brief intervention. *Journal of Happiness Studies* 9 (2): 185–196.

Mammoliti, M. (2022) 'Why boundaries should be part of your 2022 physician goals', KevinMD, 3 February. https://kevinmd.com/2022/02/why-boundaries-should-be-part-of-your-2022-physician-goals.html (accessed 16 December 2025).

Martela, F. and Pessi, A.B. (2018). Significant work is about self-realization and broader purpose: defining the key dimensions of meaningful work. *Frontiers in Psychology* 9: 363.

Mastenbroek, N.J., Jaarsma, A.D.C., Scherpbier, A.J. et al. (2014). The role of personal resources in explaining well-being and performance: A study among young veterinary professionals. *European Journal of Work and Organizational Psychology* 23 (2): 190–202.

Mastenbroek, N.J., van Beukelen, P., Demerouti, E. et al. (2015). Effects of a 1 year development programme for recently graduated veterinary professionals on personal and job resources: a combined quantitative and qualitative approach. *BMC veterinary research* 11 (1): 311.

McArthur, M., Mansfield, C., Matthew, S. et al. (2017). Resilience in veterinary students and the predictive role of mindfulness and self-compassion. *Journal of veterinary medical education* 44 (1): 106–115.

McArthur, M.L., Learey, T.J., Jarden, A. et al. (2021). Resilience of veterinarians at different career stages: the role of self-efficacy, coping strategies and personal resources for resilience in veterinary practice. *Veterinary Record* 189 (12): e771.

McIntyre, E., Lauche, R., Frawley, J. et al. (2019). Physical activity and depression symptoms in women with chronic illness and the mediating role of health-related quality of life. *Journal of affective disorders* 252: 294–299.

Moore, S.A. and O'Kell, A. (2024). Clinical research self-efficacy in academic veterinary clinicians in the United States. *Journal of the American Veterinary Medical Association* 262 (9): 1–7.

Moses, L., Malowney, M.J., and Wesley Boyd, J. (2018). Ethical conflict and moral distress in veterinary practice: A survey of North American veterinarians. *Journal of veterinary internal medicine* 32 (6): 2115–2122.

Neff, K. (2003). Self-compassion: An alternative conceptualization of a healthy attitude toward oneself. *Self and identity* 2 (2): 85–101.

Neff, K. (2011). *Self-compassion: The Proven Power of Being Kind to Yourself*. New York: Hachette UK.

Ng, B. (2018). The neuroscience of growth mindset and intrinsic motivation. *Brain Sciences* 8 (2): 2.

Noetel, M., Sanders, T., Gallardo-Gómez, D. et al. (2024). Effect of exercise for depression: systematic review and network meta-analysis of randomised controlled trials. *BMJ* 38: 1–17.

Pharris, A.B. (2025). The protective effects of hope training on the human service workforce burnout and secondary traumatic stress. *Human Service Organizations: Management, Leadership & Governance* 49 (2): 123–134.

Pohl, R., Botscharow, J., Böckelmann, I., and Thielmann, B. (2022). Stress and strain among veterinarians: a scoping review. *Irish Veterinary Journal* 75 (1): 15.

Rafiei, S., Souri, S., Nejatifar, Z., and Amerzadeh, M. (2024). The moderating role of self-efficacy in the relationship between occupational stress and mental health issues among nurses. *Scientific reports* 14 (1): 15913.

Ramos-Sanchez, C.P., Schuch, F.B., Seedat, S. et al. (2021). The anxiolytic effects of exercise for people with anxiety and related disorders: an update of the available meta-analytic evidence. *Psychiatry Research* 302: 114046.

Rohlf, V.I., Scotney, R., Monaghan, H., and Bennett, P. (2022). Predictors of professional quality of life in veterinary professionals. *Journal of Veterinary Medical Education* 49 (3): 372–381.

Salovey, P. and Mayer, J.D. (1990). Emotional intelligence. *Imagination, cognition and personality* 9 (3): 185–211.

SAMHSA "Dimensions of wellness: change your habits, change your life." SAMHSA, U.S. National Library of Medicine, 2017, Aug., pmc.ncbi.nlm.nih.gov/articles/PMC5508938/ (accessed 28 December 2024).

Samsari, E.P. and Soulis, S.G. (2019). Problem solving and resilience self-efficacy as factors of subjective well-being in Greek individuals with and without physical disabilities. *International Journal of Special Education* 33 (4): 938–953.

Selva, J. (2017) 'The history of mindfulness', PositivePsychology.com. https://positivepsychology.com/history-of-mindfulness/ (accessed 16 December 2025).

Srivastava, S., Upadhaya, P., and Jain, R. (2023). Listen to the heart or mind first? examining sequential coping mechanisms among Indians during the COVID-19 pandemic. *Frontiers in Psychology* 14: 1104973.

Swarbrick, M. (1997). A wellness model for clients. *Mental Health Special Interest Section Quarterly* 20 (1): 1–4.

Tawwab, N.G. (2021). *Set boundaries, find peace: A guide to reclaiming yourself.* New York, NY: Penguin.

Thomas, J.D. (2019). Breaching the professional–personal boundary—an unrecognized risk for burnout. *New England Journal of Medicine* 381 (11): 998–999.

Thorndike, E.L. (1920). Intelligence and its uses. *Harper's Monthly Magazine* 140: 227–235.

Troy, A.S., Wilhelm, F.H., Shallcross, A.J., and Mauss, I.B. (2010). Seeing the silver lining: cognitive reappraisal ability moderates the relationship between stress and depressive symptoms. *Emotion* 10 (6): 783–795.

Van Agteren, J., Iasiello, M., Lo, L. et al. (2021). A systematic review and meta-analysis of psychological interventions to improve mental wellbeing. *Nature human behaviour* 5 (5): 631–652.

Villani, D., Sorgente, A., Iannello, P., and Antonietti, A. (2019). The role of spirituality and religiosity in subjective well-being of individuals with different religious status. *Frontiers in Psychology* 10: 1525.

Volk, J.O., Schimmack, U., Strand, E.B. et al. (2022). Executive summary of the Merck animal health veterinarian wellbeing study III and veterinary support staff study. *Journal of the American Veterinary Medical Association* 260 (12): 1547–1553.

Wakelin, K.E., 2021. An online compassionate imagery intervention for veterinarian mental health: a feasibility study. Doctoral dissertation. University of Surrey.

Wallace, J.E. (2019). Meaningful work and well-being: a study of the positive side of veterinary work. *Veterinary Record* 185 (18): 571–571.

Wasson, R.S., Barratt, C., and O'Brien, W.H. (2020). Effects of mindfulness-based interventions on self-compassion in health care professionals: a meta-analysis. *Mindfulness* 11: 1914–1934.

Wells, J., Watson, K., Davis, R.E. et al. (2021). Associations among stress, anxiety, depression, and emotional intelligence among veterinary medicine students. *International Journal of Environmental Research and Public Health* 18 (8): 3934.

White, S.C. (2018). Veterinarians' emotional reactions and coping strategies for adverse events in spay-neuter surgical practice. *Anthrozoös* 31 (1): 117–131.

Wiest, B. (2024). This is what self-care really means, because it's not all salt baths and chocolate cake. *Thought Catalog* 4 December. https://thoughtcatalog.com/brianna-wiest/2024/04/this-is-what-self-care-really-means-because-its-not-all-salt-baths-and-chocolate-cake-2/ (accessed 28 December 2024).

Wiseman, T., Foster, K., and Curtis, K. (2016). The experience of emotional wellbeing for patients with physical injury: A qualitative follow-up study. *Injury* 47 (9): 1983–1989.

World Health Organization: WHO (2024) Self-care for health and well-being. https://www.who.int/news-room/fact-sheets/detail/self-care-health-interventions?utm_source=chatgpt.com.

Yaden, D.B., Batz-Barbarich, C.L., Ng, V. et al. (2022). A meta-analysis of religion/spirituality and life satisfaction. *Journal of Happiness Studies* 23 (8): 4147–4163.

Index